READY REFERENCE
FOR
Emergency Nursing

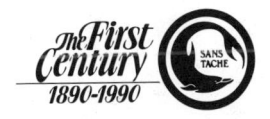

The First Century
1890-1990
SANS TACHE

READY REFERENCE FOR
Emergency Nursing

Susan Moore, RN, MS, CCRN, CEN
Clinical Nurse Specialist
Emergency Department
Washoe Medical Center
Reno, Nevada

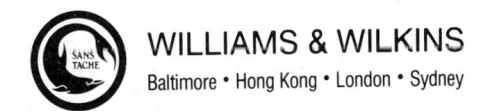

WILLIAMS & WILKINS
Baltimore • Hong Kong • London • Sydney

Editor: Susan M. Glover
Associate Editor: Majorie Kidd Keating
Copy Editors: Hilah A. Selleck, Susan Vaupel
Designer: JoAnne Janowiak
Illustration Planner: Ray Lowman
Production Coordinator: Raymond E. Reter

Copyright © 1990
Williams & Wilkins
428 East Preston Street
Baltimore, Maryland 21202, USA

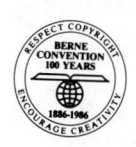

All rights reserved. This book is protected by copyright. No part of this book may be reproduced in any form or by any means, including photocopying, or utilized by any information storage and retrieval system without written permission from the copyright owner.

Accurate indications, adverse reactions, and dosage schedules for drugs are provided in this book, but it is possible that they may change. The reader is urged to review the package information data of the manufacturers of the medications mentioned.

Printed in the United States of America

Library of Congress Cataloging-in-Publication Data
Moore, Susan, 1953–
  Ready reference for emergency nursing/Susan Moore.
      p. cm.
  ISBN 0-683-06143-7
  1. Emergency nursing—Handbooks, manuals, etc. 2. Intensive care nursing—Handbooks, manuals, etc. I. Title.
  [DNLM: 1. Emergencies—nursing—handbooks. WY 39 M824r]
RT120.E4M67 1990
610.73'61—dc20
DNLM/DLC
for Library of Congress
For information about our audio products, write us at: 89-70484
Newbridge Book Clubs, 3000 Cindel Drive, Delran, NJ 08370   CIP

90 91 92 93
2 3 4 5 6 7 8 9 10

preface

If you want to learn to be an emergency nurse, this is not the book for you. This is not a "how to" textbook. It is a reference book for the practicing emergency nurse who cannot find the dopamine dosage chart or who has just been asked to put a Foley cathether into a 6-year-old. The nurse knows the effects of dopamine and knows very well how to insert a Foley, but the numbers are impossible to recall. Every emergency department has charts taped to the walls or packed into "rands" that serve as memory banks for the numbers. In this book the charts and numbers for emergency nursing have been compiled in one convenient place.

Emergency nurses must have very broad knowledge, and they are also required to make rapid, accurate decisions. Stopping to calculate a long formula is frequently impossible. In this book, the calculations are already done.

Because emergency nursing combines all of the specialties in nursing, this book by necessity is broad-ranged. The text begins with general information charts, then moves into common drug calculations. The section on laboratory values has several blanks. Laboratory values vary in different hospitals. The values that are consistently the same are listed, but the nurse will need to fill in the values that are specific to the facility in which he or she practices.

The cardiovascular section includes lead placement, basic 12-lead ECG interpretation, and other cardiac information. The nurse will not find basic rhythm interpretation. That is something that must be committed to memory. For the patient's safety, a practitioner cannot spend time looking up basic dysrhythmias.

The phone number section includes several blank pages for listing numbers specific to the setting in which the nurse practices. The pediatrics section is large because nurses in most emergency departments are not accustomed to caring for children and there are a multitude of numbers to remember.

Many of my colleagues have given me ideas for this book. I especially want to thank the nurses in the Emergency Department at Washoe Medical Center; Mary Bryant, RN; and the kind people in Medical Records.

CONTENTS

Preface v

chapter 1
GENERAL INFORMATION 1
Apothecary System to Metric System Conversion 3
Centigrade and Fahrenheit Conversion 4
Champion Trauma Score 5
C.R.A.M.S. Score 6
Estimating Dates of Confinement 6
Incubation Periods for Common Diseases 7
Laboratory Values 9
    Hematology 9
    Hemostasis 9
    Arterial Blood Gases 10
    Serum Electrolytes 10
    Enzymes 10
    Serum Hormones 11
    Lipids and Sugars 11
    Serum Protein 11
    Protein Metabolites and Pigments 11
    Urinalysis 12
    Cerebrospinal Fluid 12
Nursing Diagnosis Approved by the North American
    Nursing Diagnosis Association 13
Pounds and Kilogram Conversion 17

viii CONTENTS

chapter 2
MEDICATION REFERENCES 19
- Calculating Intravenous Drug Concentrations and Rates ... 21
- Common Intravenous Drug Concentrations (Adult) 22
- Quick Reference Dosage 24
  - Dobutamine 24
  - Dopamine 25
  - Nipride (Nitroprusside) 26
  - Nitroglycerin 27
  - Norcuron 27
- Medication Compatibility 28
- K+ Scale 29

chapter 3
CARDIOVASCULAR CARE 31
- Advanced Cardiac Life Support Algorithms 33
  - Ventricular Fibrillation and Pulseless Ventricular
    Tachycardia 33
  - Asystole (Cardiac Standstill) 36
  - Electromechanical Dissociation 37
  - Sustained Ventricular Tachycardia with a Pulse 38
  - Bradycardia (Heart rate < 60 beats/min) 40
  - Ventricular Ectopy: Acute Suppressive Therapy 41
  - Paroxysmal Supraventricular Tachycardia (PSVT) 43
- Lead Placement 44
  - Lead I 44
  - Lead II 45
  - Lead III 46
  - MCL1 47
  - Precordial (V) Leads 48
- Normal Electrocardiogram Intervals and Rate
  Determination 49
- 12-Lead ECG Interpretation 50
  - Myocardial Ischemia 50
  - Acute Injury 50
  - Myocardial Infarction 50

CONTENTS

    Digitalis Effect 51
    Strain Pattern 51
  Myocardial Infarction 51
    Anterior Myocardial Infarction 51
    Anteroseptal Myocardial Infarction 52
    Anterolateral Myocardial Infarction 52
    Inferior Myocardial Infarction 52
    Posterior Myocardial Infarction 53
    Subendocardial Myocardial Infarction 53
  Intravascular Pressures 53
  Pulmonary Artery Catheter Positions and Corresponding Waveforms 54
  Postural (Orthostatic) Blood Pressure and Pulse 54

chapter 4
PULMONARY CARE 57
  Oxygen Delivery System 59
  Abbreviations and Terms 59
  Initial Ventilator Settings 61
  Oxyhemoglobin Dissociation Curve 61

chapter 5
NEUROLOGIC CARE 63
  Glasgow Coma Scale 65
  Intracranial Pressures 65
  Dermatome Chart 67
  Cranial Nerve Testing 68
  Pupil Size Chart 69

chapter 6
ORTHOPAEDIC CARE 71
  Application of an Orthopedic Casting Laboratory (OCL) Splint 73
    Posterior Splint of Ankle (Darted) 74

x   CONTENTS

    Posterior Splint of Ankle (Reinforced) 75
    Stirrup Ankle 76
    Common Forearm and Hand Splints 77
    Boxer Splint 78
    Carpal Splint 79
    Reverse Sugar Tong 80
    Teardrop Splint 81
    Thumb Spica 82
Compartment Pressure Measurement 83

chapter 7
EYE CARE 85
Mydriatics and Miotics 87
Intraocular Pressure 88

chapter 8
TOXIC INGESTIONS 89
Toxic Dosages 91
Toxic Serum Drug Levels 91
Toxicity Nomograms 92
    Acetaminophen 92
    Ibuprofen 93
    Salicylate 94
Common Antidotes 95
Digibind Dosages 99
Cyanide Poisoning 99
Heavy Metal Chelation 100

chapter 9
BURN CARE 101
Rule of Nines 103
Lund and Browder Burn Surface Calculation 104
Fluid Replacement Formulas 105

CONTENTS **xi**

chapter 10
PEDIATRICS **107**
   Normal Vital Signs for Infants and Children 109
   Average Weight and Height for Infants and Children 109
   Equipment Guidelines according to Age and Weight 111
   Crash Drug and Defibrillation Dosages 113
   Pediatric Intravenous Drug Concentrations 113
   Formula for Intravenous Volume Replacement 114
   Modified Infant Coma Score 115
   Common Pediatric Laboratory Values 116
   Hematology 118
   Apgar Scoring 119
   Immunization Schedule 119
   Acetaminophen Dosages 121

appendix A
ABBREVIATIONS **123**

appendix B
HEALTH CARE–RELATED TELEPHONE NUMBERS **127**

chapter 1

GENERAL INFORMATION

APOTHECARY SYSTEM TO METRIC SYSTEM CONVERSION

gr xv	= 1.0	g =	1000	mg
gr x	= 0.6	g =	600	mg
gr viiss[a]	= 0.5	g =	500	mg
gr v	= .30	g =	300	mg
gr iii	= 0.2	g =	200	mg
gr 1½	= 0.1	g =	100	mg
gr 1	= 0.06	g =	60	mg
gr 3/4	= 0.05	g =	50	mg
gr 1/2	= 0.03	g =	30	mg
gr 1/4	= 0.015	g =	15	mg
gr 1/6	= 0.010	g =	10	mg
gr 1/8	= 0.008	g =	8	mg
gr 1/12	= 0.005	g =	5	mg
gr 1/15	= 0.004	g =	4	mg
gr 1/20	= 0.0032	g =	3	mg
gr 1/30	= 0.0022	g =	2	mg
gr 1/40	= 0.0015	g =	1.5	mg
gr 1/50	= 0.0012	g =	1.2	mg
gr 1/60	= 0.001	g =	1	mg
gr 1/100	= 0.0006	g =	0.6	mg
gr 1/120	= 0.0005	g =	0.5	mg
gr 1/150	= 0.0004	g =	0.4	mg
gr 1/200	= 0.0003	g =	0.3	mg
gr 1/300	= 0.0002	g =	0.2	mg
gr 1/600	= 0.0001	g =	0.1	mg

[a]ss = ½.

CENTIGRADE AND FAHRENHEIT CONVERSION

Formula for converting centigrade to Fahrenheit:

$$(C \times 9/5) + 32 = F$$

Formula for converting Fahrenheit to centigrade:

$$(F - 32) \times 5/9 = C$$

C	F	C	F	C	F	C	F
0.0	32.0	34.8	94.6	36.9	98.4	38.7	101.7
26.6	80.0	35.0	95.0	37.0	98.6	38.8	101.8
27.2	81.0	35.2	95.4	37.1	98.8	38.9	102.0
27.7	82.0	35.4	95.7	37.2	99.0	39.0	102.2
28.3	83.0	35.5	95.9	37.3	99.1	39.1	102.4
28.9	84.0	35.6	96.1	37.4	99.3	39.2	102.6
29.4	85.0	35.7	96.3	37.5	99.5	39.3	102.7
30.0	86.0	35.8	96.4	37.6	99.6	39.4	102.9
30.5	87.0	35.9	96.6	37.7	99.8	39.5	103.1
31.1	88.0	36.0	96.8	37.8	100.0	39.6	103.3
31.7	89.0	36.1	96.9	37.9	100.2	39.7	103.5
32.2	90.0	36.2	97.2	38.0	100.4	39.8	103.6
32.8	91.0	36.3	97.3	38.1	100.6	39.9	103.8
33.3	92.0	36.4	97.5	38.2	100.8	40.0	104.0
34.0	93.2	36.5	97.7	38.3	100.9	40.6	105.0
34.2	93.6	36.6	97.9	38.4	101.1	41.1	106.0
34.4	93.9	36.7	98.0	38.5	101.3	41.7	107.0
34.6	94.3	36.8	98.2	38.6	101.5	100	212

CHAMPION TRAUMA SCORE[a]

Each parameter is assigned a number. The Glasgow Coma Score is totaled, then converted to scale points. The numbers given to each parameter are totaled. The lower the total number, the greater the severity of injury. The lowest score is 1, the highest is 16.

Respiratory Rate			Glasgow Coma Scale	
10–24 min	4		Eye Opening	
24–35/min	3		Spontaneous	4
36/min or greater	2		To voice	3
1–9/min	1		To pain	2
None	0		None	1
Respiratory Expansion			Verbal Response	
Normal	1		Oriented	5
Retractive	0		Confused	4
Systolic Blood Pressure			Inappropriate words	3
90 mm Hg or greater	4		Incomprehensible words	2
70–89 mm Hg	3		None	1
50–69 mm Hg	2		Motor Response	
0–49 mm Hg	1		Obeys command	6
No pulse	0		Localizes to pain	5
Capillary Refill			Withdraws from pain	4
Normal	2		Flexion to pain	3
Delayed	1		Extension to pain	2
None	0		None	1

Total Glasgow Coma Scale Points:
    14–15 = 5
    11–13 = 4
      8–10 = 3
      5–7 = 2
      3–4 = 1

Total Trauma Score   1–16

---

[a]From Champion HR, Sacco WJ, Carnazzo AJ, Copes W, Fouty WJ. Trauma score. *Crit Care Med* 1981; 9(9): 672–676. Williams & Wilkins.

C.R.A.M.S. SCORE

Circulation	Normal capillary refill and BP more than 100	2
	Delayed capillary refill or BP 85 to 100	1
	No capillary refill or BP less than 85	0
Respirations	Normal	2
	Abnormal (labored or shallow)	1
	Absent	0
Abdomen	Abdomen or thorax nontender	2
	Abdomen or thorax tender	1
	Abdomen rigid, flail chest, or penetrating wounds to abdomen or thorax	0
Motor	Normal	2
	Responds to pain only (other than decerebrate)	1
	No response (or decerebrate)	0
Speech	Normal	2
	Confused	1
	No intelligible words	0
Total		—

A score equal to or less than 8 is major trauma. A score equal to or more than 9 is minor trauma.

ESTIMATING DATES OF CONFINEMENT

To obtain estimated date of delivery (EDC) add 7 days to date of last menstrual period (LMP), then subtract 3 months.

LMP	EDC	LMP	EDC	LMP	EDC
Jan 1	Oct 8	Feb 12	Nov 19	Mar 26	Jan 2
Jan 8	Oct 15	Feb 19	Nov 26	Apr 2	Jan 9
Jan 15	Oct 22	Feb 26	Dec 5	Apr 9	Jan 16
Jan 22	Oct 29	Mar 5	Dec 12	Apr 16	Jan 23
Jan 29	Nov 5	Mar 12	Dec 19	Apr 23	Jan 30
Feb 5	Nov 12	Mar 19	Dec 26	Apr 30	Feb 7

ESTIMATING DATES OF CONFINEMENT *(cont.)*

To obtain estimated date of delivery (EDC) add 7 days to date of last menstrual period (LMP), then subtract 3 months.

LMP	EDC	LMP	EDC	LMP	EDC
May 7	Feb 14	Jul 30	May 6	Oct 22	Jul 29
May 14	Feb 21	Aug 6	May 13	Oct 29	Aug 5
May 21	Feb 28	Aug 13	May 20	Nov 5	Aug 12
May 28	Mar 4	Aug 20	May 27	Nov 12	Aug 19
Jun 4	Mar 11	Aug 27	Jun 3	Nov 19	Aug 26
Jun 11	Mar 18	Sep 3	Jun 10	Nov 26	Sep 3
Jun 18	Mar 25	Sep 10	Jun 17	Dec 3	Sep 10
Jun 25	Apr 2	Sep 17	Jun 24	Dec 10	Sep 17
Jul 2	Apr 9	Sep 24	Jul 1	Dec 17	Sep 24
Jul 9	Apr 16	Oct 1	Jul 8	Dec 24	Oct 1
Jul 16	Apr 23	Oct 8	Jul 15		
Jul 23	Apr 30	Oct 15	Jul 22		

INCUBATION PERIODS FOR COMMON DISEASES

Disease	Incubation Period	Comments
Bubonic plague	2–6 days	
Botulism	6 hr–8 days	
Common cold	1–3 days	
Chicken pox (Varicella)	13–17 days	Can return to school when a few scabs remain
Conjunctivitis		Can return to school 24 hr after antibiotics begun
Diphtheria	3–7 days	
Food poisoning (*Staphylococcus aureus*)	1–6 hr	Symptoms subside in 18 hr
Herpes simplex	2–12 days	

INCUBATION PERIODS FOR COMMON DISEASES *(cont.)*

Disease	Incubation Period	Comments
Impetigo		Can return to school 24 hr after antibiotics begun
Influenza	24–48 hr	
Lyme disease	2 days–5 wk	Rash may not be present in every case
Malaria	12–30 days	
Mononucleosis	Children—10 days Adults—30–50 days	
Mumps	14–25 days	
Pertussis (whooping cough)	7–10 days	
Polio	5–35 days	
Rabies	1–3 mo	
Respiratory syncytial virus	4–5 days	
Rocky Mountain spotted fever	2–14 days	
Roseola	10–15 days	
Rubella (German measles)	16–18 days	Can return to school 6 days after rash appears
Rubeola (measles)	10–14 days	Can return to school 6 days after rash appears
Scarlet fever	2–5 days	
Shigellosis	1–4 days	
Strep throat	1–5 days	
Tetanus	2–10 days	
Tick fever	4–5 days	

LABORATORY VALUES

(See Chapter 10 for pediatric laboratory values)

Hematology
  Basophils: Relative to WBC count: 0.3–2%
          Absolute: 12–200/μl
  Eosinophils: Relative to WBC count: 0.3–7%
          Absolute: 12–760/μl
  Erythrocyte sedimentation rate (ESR): Females: 0–20 mm/hr
                                        Males: 0–10 mm/hr
  Hematocrit (HCT): Females: _____

                    Males: _____
  Hemoglobin (Hgb) (venous sample): Females: _____

                                    Males: _____
  Lymphocytes: Relative to WBC count: 16.2–43%
          Absolute: 660–4,600/μl
  Mean corpuscular hemoglobin (MCH): 26–32
  Mean corpuscular hemoglobin concentration (MCHC): 30–36%
  Mean corpuscular volume (MCV): 84–99
  Monocytes: Relative to WBC count: 0.6–9.6%
          Absolute: 24–960/μl
  Neutrophils: Relative to WBC count: 47.6–76.8%
          Absolute: 1,950–8,400/μl
  Red blood cell (RBC) count: Females: 4.2–5.4 million/μl
                              Males: 4.5–6.2 million/μl
  Reticulocyte count: 0.5–2.0% of total RBC count
  Serum iron: Females: 80–150 μg/dl
          Males: 70–150 μg/dl
  Total iron binding capacity: Females: 300–450 μg/dl
                               Males: 300–400 μg/dl
  White blood cell (WBC) count: 4,100–10,900/μl
Hemostasis
  Activated partial thromboplastin time (APTT): 25–36 sec

  Bleeding time: _____
  Clotting time (whole blood): 5–15 min

LABORATORY VALUES *(cont.)*

(See Chapter 10 for pediatric laboratory values)

Fibrin split products: _____

Plasma fibrinogen: _____
Plasma thrombin time (thrombin clotting time): _____
Platelet count: 130,000–370,000/ml

Prothrombin time (PT): _____ (Patients on oral anticoagulants should be between 1½ to 2 times normal.)

Arterial blood gases

Arterial carbon dioxide pressure ($PaCO_2$): 35–45 mm Hg

Arterial oxygen pressure (PaO_2): _____

Bicarbonate (HCO_3): 22–26 mEq/liter

Oxygen content (O_2CT): _____

Oxygen saturation (O_2Sat): _____

pH: 7.35–7.42

Electrolytes, serum
 Calcium: _____
 Chloride: 100–108 mEq/liter

 Magnesium: _____

 Phosphates: _____
 Potassium: 3.8–5.5 mEq/liter
 Sodium: 135–145 mEq/liter

Enzymes
 Acid phosphatase: _____

 Alkaline phosphatase: _____

 Creatinine phosphokinase (CPK), total: Women: 15–57 u/liter
 Men: 23–99 u/liter

 CPK-BB: 0
 CPK-MB: 0–7 IU/liter

LABORATORY VALUES *(cont.)*

(See Chapter 10 for pediatric laboratory values)

CPK-MM: 5–70 IU/liter
Lactic dehydrogenase (LDH), total: 48–115 IU/liter
LDH1: 18.1–29% of total
LDH2: 29.4–37.5% of total
Serum glutamic-oxaloacetic transaminase (SGOT): 8–20 u/liter
Serum glutamic-pyruvic transaminase (SGPT): Women: 9–24 u/liter
                                                       Men: 10–32 u/liter

Serum amylase: _____

Serum lipase: _____

Hormones, serum
    Human chorionic gonadotropin (HCG): 0–3 mIU/ml in nonpregnant women
    Thyroxine (T_4): _____

    Triiodothyronine (T_3): _____

Sugars and Lipids
    Fasting blood glucose: 70–100 mg/100 ml blood
    Total cholesterol: 120–330 mg/dl (American Heart Association recommends a total cholesterol level less than 200 mg/dl)
    Two-hour postprandial plasma glucose: 70–145 mg/100 ml blood

Protein, Serum
    α_1-globulin: 0.1–0.4 g/dl
    α_2-globulin: 0.5–1.0 g/dl
    β-globulin: 0.7–1.2 g/dl
    γ-globulin: 0.5–1.6 g/dl
    Albumin fraction: 3.3–4.5 g/dl
    Total protein: 6.6–7.9 g/dl

Protein metabolites and pigments
    Blood urea nitrogen (BUN): 8–20 mg/dl
    Direct serum bilirubin: 0–0.5 mg/dl
    Indirect serum bilirubin: 0–1.1 mg/dl
    Plasma ammonia: 0–50 µg/dl

LABORATORY VALUES (cont.)

(See Chapter 10 for pediatric laboratory values)

Serum creatine: Females: 0.6–1.0 mg/dl
　　　　　　　　Males: 0.2–0.6 mg/dl
Serum creatinine: Females: 0.6–0.9 mg/dl
　　　　　　　　　Males: 0.8–1.2 mg/dl
Serum uric acid: Females: 2.3–6.0 mg/dl
　　　　　　　　　Males: 4.3–8.0 mg/dl

Urinalysis
　Casts: None, except occasional hyaline casts
　Crystals: Present
　Epithelial cells: Few
　Glucose: None
　Ketones: None
　Parasites: None
　pH: 4.5–8
　Protein: None
　RBCs: 0–3 per high-power field
　Specific gravity: 1.025–1.030
　WBCs: 0–4 per high-power field
　Yeast cells: None

Cerebrospinal fluid
　Appearance: Clear, colorless
　Chloride: 118–130 mEq/liter
　γ-globulin: 3–12% of total protein
　Glucose: 50–80 mg/100 ml (⅔ of blood glucose)
　Pressure: 50–180 mm H_2O
　Protein: 15–45 mg/100 ml
　RBCs: None
　WBCs: 0–5

NURSING DIAGNOSES APPROVED BY THE NORTH AMERICAN NURSING DIAGNOSIS ASSOCIATION[a]

Pattern 1: Exchanging

1.1.2.1	Altered nutrition: More than body requirements
1.1.2.2	Altered nutrition: Less than body requirements
1.1.2.3	Altered Nutrition: Potential for more than body requirements
1.2.1.1	Potential for infection
1.2.2.1	Potential for altered body temperature
1.2.2.2	Hypothermia
1.2.2.3	Hyperthermia
1.2.2.4	Ineffective thermoregulation
1.2.3.1	Dysreflexia
1.3.1.1	Constipation
1.3.1.1.1	Perceived constipation
1.3.1.1.2	Colonic constipation
1.3.1.2	Diarrhea
1.3.1.3	Bowel incontinence
1.3.2	Altered urinary elimination
1.3.2.1.1	Stress incontinence
1.3.2.1.2	Reflex incontinence
1.3.2.1.3	Urge incontinence
1.3.2.1.4	Functional incontinence
1.3.2.1.5	Total incontinence
1.3.2.2	Urinary retention
1.4.1.1	Altered (*specify type*) tissue perfusion (renal, cerebral, cardiopulmonary, gastrointestinal, peripheral)
1.4.1.2.1	Fluid volume excess
1.4.1.2.2.1	Fluid volume deficit
1.4.1.2.2.2	Potential fluid volume deficit
1.4.2.1	Decreased cardiac output
1.5.1.1	Impaired gas exchange
1.5.1.2	Ineffective airway clearance
1.5.1.3	Ineffective breathing pattern

NURSING DIAGNOSES APPROVED BY THE NORTH AMERICAN NURSING DIAGNOSIS ASSOCIATION[a] (cont.)

1.6.1	Potential for injury
1.6.1.1	Potential for suffocation
1.6.1.2	Potential for poisoning
1.6.1.3	Potential for trauma
1.6.1.4	Potential for aspiration
1.6.1.5	Potential for disuse syndrome
1.6.2.1	Impaired tissue integrity
1.6.2.1.1	Altered oral mucous membrane
1.6.2.1.2.1	Impaired skin integrity
1.6.2.1.2.2	Potential impaired skin integrity

Pattern 2: Communicating

2.1.1.1	Impaired verbal communication

Pattern 3: Relating

3.1.1	Impaired social interaction
3.1.2	Social isolation
3.2.1	Altered role performance
3.2.1.1.1	Altered parenting
3.2.1.1.2	Potential altered parenting
3.2.1.2.1	Sexual dysfunction
3.2.2	Altered family processes
3.2.3.1	Parental role conflict
3.3	Altered sexuality patterns

Pattern 4: Valuing

4.1.1	Spiritual distress (distress of the human spirit)

Pattern 5: Choosing

5.1.1.1	Ineffective individual coping
5.1.1.1.1	Impaired adjustment
5.1.1.1.2	Defensive coping
5.1.1.1.3	Ineffective denial
5.1.2.1.1	Ineffective family coping: disabling
5.1.2.1.2	Ineffective family coping: compromised
5.1.2.2	Family coping: potential for growth
5.2.1.1	Noncompliance (*specify*)
5.3.1.1	Decisional conflict (*specify*)
5.4	Health-seeking behaviors (*specify*)

NURSING DIAGNOSES APPROVED BY THE NORTH AMERICAN NURSING DIAGNOSIS ASSOCIATION[a] *(cont.)*

Pattern 6: Moving
- 6.1.1.1   Impaired physical mobility
- 6.1.1.2   Activity intolerance
- 6.1.1.2.1   Fatigue
- 6.1.1.3   Potential activity intolerance
- 6.2.1   Sleep pattern disturbance
- 6.3.1.1   Diversional activity deficit
- 6.4.1.1   Impaired home maintenance management
- 6.4.2   Altered health maintenance
- 6.5.1   Feeding self-care deficit
- 6.5.1.1   Impaired swallowing
- 6.5.1.2   Ineffective breastfeeding
- 6.5.2   Bathing/hygiene self-care deficit
- 6.5.3   Dressing/grooming self-care deficit
- 6.5.4   Toileting self-care deficit
- 6.6   Altered growth and development

Pattern 7: Perceiving
- 7.1.1   Body image disturbance
- 7.1.2   Self-esteem disturbance
- 7.1.2.1   Chronic low self-esteem
- 7.1.2.2   Situational low self-esteem
- 7.1.3   Personal identity disturbance
- 7.2   Sensory/perceptual alterations (*specify*) (visual, auditory, kinesthetic, gustatory, tactile, olfactory)
- 7.2.1.1   Unilateral neglect
- 7.3.1   Hopelessness
- 7.3.2   Powerlessness

Pattern 8: Knowing
- 8.1.1   Knowledge deficit (*specify*)
- 8.3   Altered thought processes

Pattern 9: Feeling
- 9.1.1   Pain
- 9.1.1.1   Chronic pain
- 9.2.1.1   Dysfunctional grieving
- 9.2.1.2   Anticipatory grieving

NURSING DIAGNOSES APPROVED BY THE NORTH AMERICAN NURSING DIAGNOSIS ASSOCIATION[a] *(cont.)*

9.2.2	Potential for violence: self-directed or directed at others
9.2.3	Posttrauma response
9.2.3.1	Rape-trauma syndrome
9.2.3.1.1	Rape-trauma syndrome: compound reaction
9.2.3.1.2	Rape-trauma syndrome: silent reaction
9.3.1	Anxiety
9.3.2	Fear

[a]From the North American Nursing Diagnosis Association.

POUND AND KILOGRAM CONVERSION

$1 \text{ kg} = 2.2 \text{ lb}$

Numbers in the farthest left column are in increments of 10 lb. Numbers going across the top are in increments of 1 lb. Intersect the two to get the equivalent in kilograms. Example: 196 lb is 88.9 kg.

lb	0	1	2	3	4	5	6	7	8	9
0	0	0.45	0.9	1.36	1.81	2.26	2.72	3.17	3.62	4.08
10	4.53	4.98	5.44	5.89	6.35	6.80	7.25	7.71	8.16	8.61
20	9.07	9.52	9.97	10.43	10.88	11.34	11.79	12.24	12.7	13.15
30	13.6	14.06	14.51	14.96	15.42	15.87	16.32	16.78	17.23	17.69
40	18.14	18.59	19.05	19.5	19.95	20.41	20.86	21.31	21.77	22.22
50	22.68	23.13	23.58	24.04	24.49	24.94	25.4	25.85	26.3	26.76
60	27.21	27.66	28.12	28.57	29.03	29.48	29.93	30.39	30.84	31.29
70	31.75	32.20	32.65	33.11	33.56	34.02	34.47	34.92	35.38	35.83
80	36.28	36.74	37.19	37.64	38.1	38.55	39	39.46	39.91	40.37
90	40.82	41.27	41.73	42.18	42.63	43.09	43.54	43.99	44.45	44.9
100	45.36	45.81	46.26	46.72	47.17	47.62	48.08	48.53	48.98	49.44
110	49.89	50.34	50.8	51.25	51.71	52.16	52.61	53.07	53.52	53.97
120	54.43	54.88	55.33	55.79	56.24	56.7	57.15	57.6	58.06	58.51
130	58.96	59.42	59.87	60.32	60.78	61.23	61.68	62.14	62.59	63.05
140	63.5	63.95	64.41	64.86	65.31	65.77	66.22	66.67	67.13	67.58
150	68.04	68.49	68.94	69.4	69.85	70.30	70.76	71.21	71.66	72.12
160	72.57	73.02	73.48	73.93	74.39	74.84	75.29	75.75	76.20	76.65
170	77.11	77.56	78.01	78.47	78.92	79.38	79.83	80.28	80.74	81.19

POUND AND KILOGRAM CONVERSION

1 kg = 2.2 lb

Numbers in the farthest left column are in increments of 10 lb. Numbers going across the top are in increments of 1 lb. Intersect the two to get the equivalent in kilograms. Example: 196 lb is 88.9 kg.

lb	0	1	2	3	4	5	6	7	8	9
180	81.64	82.1	82.55	83	83.46	83.91	84.36	84.82	85.27	85.73
190	86.18	86.68	87.09	87.54	87.99	88.45	88.9	89.35	89.81	90.26
200	90.72	91.17	91.62	92.08	92.53	92.98	93.44	93.89	94.34	94.8
210	95.45	95.91	96.36	96.82	97.27	97.73	98.18	98.64	99.09	99.55

chapter 2

MEDICATION REFERENCES

CALCULATING INTRAVENOUS DRUG CONCENTRATIONS AND RATES

To determine micrograms per milliliter:

$$\frac{ml}{mg} \times 1000 = \mu g/ml$$

To determine micrograms per kilogram per minute being received when volume rate (milliliters per hour) is known:

$$\frac{\mu g/ml \times ml/min}{\text{patient's weight in kg}} = \mu g/kg/min$$

To determine volume rate (milliliters per hour) when micrograms per kilogram per minute desired is known:

$$\frac{\text{patient's weight in kg} \times \mu g/kg/min}{\mu g/ml} \times 60 = ml/hr$$

For standard microdrip tubing, gtts/min = ml/hr

COMMON INTRAVENOUS DRUG CONCENTRATIONS (ADULT)

Drug	Add	To	Final Concentration
Aminocaproic acid (Amicar)	30 g (120 ml)	380 ml D5W	60 mg/ml
Aminophylline	1 g (40 ml)	500 ml D5W	2 mg/ml
Amrinone (Inocar)	200 mg (40 ml)	160 ml NS	1 mg/ml
Bretylium (Bretylol)	1 g (20 ml)	250 ml D5W	4 mg/ml
Dobutamine (Dobutrex)	250 mg (20 ml)	250 ml D5W	1000 µg/ml
Dopamine (Intropin)	400 mg (5 ml)	250 ml D5W	1600 µg/ml
Dopamine Double Strength	800 mg (10 ml)	250 ml D5W	3200 µg/ml
Epinephrine	2 mg (20 ml)	250 ml D5W	8 µg/ml
Esmolol (Brevibloc)	2.5 g (10 ml)	250 ml D5W	10 mg/ml
Heparin	25,000 U	500 ml D5W	50 U/ml
Insulin	62.5 U	250 ml NS	0.25 U/ml (4 ml/unit)
Isoproterenol (Isuprel)	1 mg (5 ml)	500 ml D5W	2 µg/ml
Labetalol (Trandate)	200 mg (40 ml)	160 ml D5W	1 mg/ml
Lidocaine (Xylocaine)	2 g (10 ml)	500 ml D5W	4 mg/ml
Nitroglycerine (Tridil)	50 mg (10 ml)	250 ml D5W (glass)	200 µg/ml
Nitroprusside (Nipride)	50 mg	250 ml D5W	200 µg/ml
Norepinephrine (Levophed)	4 mg (4 ml)	250 ml D5W	16 µg/ml
Midazolam (Versed)	25 mg (25 ml)	250 ml D5W	1 mg/12 ml
Phenylephrine (Neo-Synephrine)	10 mg (1 ml)	250 ml D5W	40 µg/ml

COMMON INTRAVENOUS DRUG CONCENTRATIONS (ADULT) (cont.)

Drug	Add	To	Final Concentration
Procainamide (Pronestyl)	2 g (20 ml)	500 ml D5W	4 mg/ml
Propranolol (Inderal)	10 mg (10 ml)	250 ml D5W	40 µg/ml
Tissue Plasminogen Activator (TPA)	100 mg	100 ml water	1 mg/ml
Vasopressin (Pitressin)	100 U (5 ml)	500 ml D5W	0.2 U/ml
Verapamil (Isoptin)	100 mg (40 ml)	60 ml D5W	1000 µg/ml
Vecuronium (Norcuron)	30 mg	500 ml D5W	50 µg/ml

QUICK REFERENCE DOSAGE

DOBUTAMINE, ml/hr

250 mg in 250 ml D5W = 1,000 μg/ml

Desired Dose, μg/kg/min	Body weight, lb (kg)													
	99 (45)	110 (50)	121 (55)	132 (60)	143 (65)	154 (70)	165 (75)	176 (80)	187 (85)	198 (90)	208 (95)	220 (100)	231 (105)	242 (110)
1	3	3	3	4	4	4	5	5	5	5	5	6	6	7
2.5	7	8	9	9	10	11	11	12	13	14	14	15	16	17
5	14	15	17	18	20	21	23	24	26	27	29	30	32	33
7.5	20	23	25	27	29	32	34	36	38	41	43	45	47	50
10	27	30	33	35	39	42	45	48	51	54	57	60	63	66
12.5	34	39	41	45	49	53	56	60	64	68	71	75	79	83
15	41	45	50	54	59	63	68	73	77	81	86	90	95	99
20	54	60	65	72	78	84	90	95	102	108	114	120	126	132

DOPAMINE, μg/kg/min

400 mg in 250 ml D5W = 1600 μg/ml

	Body weight, lb (kg)													
ml/hr	99 (45)	110 (50)	121 (55)	132 (60)	143 (65)	154 (70)	165 (75)	176 (80)	187 (85)	198 (90)	209 (95)	220 (100)	231 (105)	242 (110)
5	2.9	2.6	2.4	2.2	2	1.9	1.8	1.6	1.55	1.5	1.4	1.3	1.25	1.2
10	5.9	5.3	4.9	4.5	4.1	3.8	3.6	3.3	3.1	3	2.8	2.7	2.5	2.4
15	8.9	8	7.3	6.6	6.1	5.7	5.3	5	4.7	4.4	4.2	4	3.8	3.6
20	11.8	10.7	9.7	8.9	8.2	7.6	7.1	6.7	6.3	5.9	5.6	5.3	5.1	4.9
25	14.8	13.4	12.1	11.1	10.2	9.5	8.9	8.4	7.8	7.4	7	6.6	6.3	6
30	17.8	16	14.6	13.3	12.3	11.4	10.7	10	9.4	8.9	8.4	8	7.6	7.3
35	20.7	18.6	17	15.5	14.3	13.3	12.4	11.6	11	10.3	9.8	9.3	8.9	8.5
40	23.7	21.3	19.4	17.8	16.4	15.2	14.2	13.3	12.6	11.9	11.2	10.7	10.2	9.7
45	26.6	24	21.8	20	18.4	17.1	16	15	14.1	13.3	12.6	12	11.4	10.9
50	29.6	26.7	24.2	22.2	20.5	19	17.8	16.7	15.7	14.8	14	13.3	12.7	12.1
55	32.6	29.3	26.6	24.4	22.5	20.9	19.5	18.3	17.2	16.3	15.4	14.6	13.9	13.3
60	35.6	32	29.1	26.7	24.6	22.9	21.3	20	18.8	17.8	16.8	16	15.2	14.6
70	41.5	37.3	34	31.1	28.7	26.7	24.9	23.3	22	20.7	19.6	18.7	17.8	17
80	47.4	42.7	38.8	35.6	32.8	30.5	28.4	26.7	25.1	23.7	22.5	21.3	20.3	19.4
90	53.3	48	43.6	40	36.9	34.3	32	30	28.2	26.7	25.3	24	22.9	21.8
100	59.3	53.3	48.5	44.5	41	38.1	35.6	33.3	31.4	29.6	28.1	26.7	25.4	24.3

NIPRIDE (NITROPRUSSIDE), ml/hr

50 mg in 250 ml D5W = 200 µg/ml[a]

Desired Dose, µg/kg/min	Body weight, lb (kg)															
	88 (40)	99 (45)	110 (50)	121 (55)	132 (60)	143 (65)	154 (70)	165 (75)	176 (80)	187 (85)	198 (90)	208 (95)	220 (100)	231 (105)	242 (110)
0.5	6	7	8	8	9	10	11	11	12	13	14	14	15	16	16
1	12	14	15	17	18	20	21	23	24	26	27	29	30	32	33
2	24	27	30	33	36	39	42	45	48	51	54	57	60	63	66
3	36	41	45	50	54	59	63	68	73	77	81	86	90	95	99
4	48	54	60	66	72	78	84	90	96	102	108	114	120	126	132
5	60	68	75	83	90	98	105	113	120	128	135	143	150	157	165
6	72	81	90	99	108	117	126	135	144	153	162	171	180	189	198
7	84	95	105	116	126	137	147	158	168	179	189	200	210	220	231
8	96	108	120	132	144	156	168	180	192	204	216	228	240	252	264
9	108	122	135	148	162	176	189	203	216	230	243	256	270	283	297
10	120	135	150	165	180	195	210	225	240	255	270	285	300	315	330

[a]Note: If you double the concentration by adding 100 mg to 250 ml D5W, divide the milliliters per hour by 2.

NITROGLYCERIN[a]

50 mg in 250 ml D5W (glass or special bottle)

1.5	ml/hr	=	5 μg/min	21	ml/hr	=	70 μg/min
3	ml/hr	=	10 μg/min	24	ml/hr	=	80 μg/min
4.5	ml/hr	=	15 μg/min	27	ml/hr	=	90 μg/min
6	ml/hr	=	20 μg/min	30	ml/hr	=	100 μg/min
9	ml/hr	=	30 μg/min	33	ml/hr	=	110 μg/min
12	ml/hr	=	40 μg/min	36	ml/hr	=	120 μg/min
15	ml/hr	=	50 μg/min	39	ml/hr	=	130 μg/min
18	ml/hr	=	60 μg/min	42	ml/hr	=	140 μg/min

[a]Use special nitroglycerin i.v. tubing.

QUICK REFERENCE NORCURON (VECURONIUM) DOSAGE[a]

30 mg in 500 ml D5W = 60 μg/ml

_____ kg × 1.0 = _____ ml/hr = 1.0 μg/kg/min

_____ kg × 0.92 = _____ ml/hr = 0.92 μg/kg/min

_____ kg × 0.83 = _____ ml/hr = 0.83 μg/kg/min

_____ kg × 0.75 = _____ ml/hr = 0.75 μg/kg/min

_____ kg × 0.67 = _____ ml/hr = 0.67 μg/kg/min

_____ kg × 0.58 = _____ ml/hr = 0.58 μg/kg/min

_____ kg × 0.50 = _____ ml/hr = 0.50 μg/kg/min

_____ kg × 0.42 = _____ ml/hr = 0.42 μg/kg/min

_____ kg × 0.33 = _____ ml/hr = 0.33 μg/kg/min

_____ kg × 0.25 = _____ ml/hr = 0.25 μg/kg/min

_____ kg × 0.16 = _____ ml/hr = 0.16 μg/kg/min

_____ kg × 0.08 = _____ ml/hr = 0.08 μg/kg/min

[a]Formula: Ideal body weight in kg × dosing factor = ml/hr = μg/kg/min

READY REFERENCE FOR EMERGENCY NURSING

Drug Compatibility Chart

Column legend (left to right):
1. Verapamil (Isoptin)
2. Propanolol HCl (Inderal)
3. Procainamide HCl (Pronestyl)
4. Potassium Chloride
5. Phenytoin Sodium (Dilantin)
6. Norepinephrine (Levophed)
7. Nitroprusside Sodium (Nipride)
8. Nitroglycerine
9. Morphine Sulfate
10. Meperidine HCl (Demerol)
11. Magnesium Sulfate
12. Lidocaine HCl (Xylocaine)
13. Isoproterenol Isuprel
14. Insulin Regular
15. Heparin Sodium
16. Furosemide (Lasix)
17. Epinephrine
18. Dopamine HCl (Intropin)
19. Dobutamine HCl (Dobutrex)
20. Diphenhydramine HCl (Benadryl)
21. Digoxin (Lanoxin)
22. Diazepam (Valium)
23. Cimetidine (Tagamet)
24. Bretylium Tosylate (Bretylol)
25. Atropine Sulfate
26. Aminophylline

Drug	1	2	3	4	5	6	7	8	9	10	11	12	13	14	15	16	17	18	19	20	21	22	23	24	25	26
Aminophylline	C	U	U	C	I	I	I	I	I	U	U	C	U	I	C	U	I	C	I	U	U	I	U	C	U	—
Atropine Sulfate	U	U	I	U	U	U	I	I	C	C	U	U	U	U	U	U	U	C	C	U	I	C	U	U	—	U
Bretylium Tosylate (Bretylol)	C	U	C	C	U	U	I	C	C	C	U	C	U	U	U	U	U	C	C	U	U	I	U	—	U	C
Cimetidine (Tagamet)	C	U	U	C	U	C	I	I	U	U	U	C	C	C	U	C	C	U	U	U	C	I	—	U	C	U
Diazepam (Valium)	I	I	I	I	I	I	I	I	I	I	I	I	I	I	I	I	I	I	I	I	I	—	I	I	I	I
Digoxin (Lanoxin)	C	I	U	S	U	U	I	I	U	U	U	C	U	U	S	U	U	U	I	U	—	I	C	U	U	U
Diphenhydramine HCl (Benadryl)	U	U	U	U	I	U	I	I	C	C	U	C	U	U	U	I	U	U	U	—	U	I	U	U	C	U
Dobutamine HCl (Dobutrex)	U	C	C	C	I	C	I	I	C	U	I	C	C	I	I	I	C	C	—	U	I	I	U	C	C	I
Dopamine HCl (Intropin)	C	U	U	C	U	U	I	I	U	U	U	C	U	U	C	U	U	C	—	U	U	I	U	C	U	C
Epinephrine	C	U	U	S	U	U	I	I	U	U	U	U	U	U	S	U	U	—	U	C	U	I	C	U	U	I
Furosemide (Lasix)	C	U	U	S	U	U	I	I	U	I	U	U	U	S	U	U	—	U	I	I	U	I	C	U	U	U
Heparin Sodium	C	U	C	C	I	C	I	I	I	C	C	C	C	C	S	—	S	C	I	U	S	I	U	U	U	C
Insulin Regular	C	U	U	C	U	I	U	U	C	C	U	C	U	U	—	C	U	U	U	I	U	U	I	C	U	U	I
Isoproterenol Isuprel	C	I	U	C	U	U	I	I	U	U	U	I	U	—	U	C	U	U	U	C	U	U	I	C	U	U	U
Lidocaine HCl (Xylocaine)	C	U	C	C	I	U	I	I	U	U	U	—	I	C	C	U	U	C	C	C	I	C	C	U	C
Magnesium Sulfate	C	U	U	C	U	C	I	I	U	U	—	U	U	C	C	U	U	U	I	U	U	U	I	U	U	U
Meperidine HCl (Demerol)	U	U	U	U	U	I	I	I	—	U	U	U	U	I	U	U	U	C	U	I	U	C	C	U
Morphine Sulfate	U	U	U	U	I	U	I	I	—	I	U	U	U	U	I	U	U	U	C	C	U	I	U	C	C	I
Nitroglycerine	I	I	I	I	I	I	—	I	I	I	I	I	I	I	I	I	I	I	I	I	I	I	I	I	I	I
Nitroprusside Sodium (Nipride)	I	I	I	I	I	I	—	I	I	I	I	I	I	I	I	I	I	I	I	I	I	I	I	I	I	I
Norepinephrine (Levophed)	C	U	U	C	I	—	I	I	U	U	C	U	U	U	C	U	U	U	C	U	U	I	C	U	U	I
Phenytoin Sodium (Dilantin)	C	U	I	U	—	I	I	I	I	U	U	I	U	I	I	U	U	U	I	U	I	U	U	U	I
Potassium Chloride	U	U	U	—	U	C	I	I	U	U	C	C	C	C	S	S	C	C	U	S	I	C	C	U	C
Procainamide HCl (Pronestyl)	C	U	—	U	I	U	I	I	U	U	U	C	U	U	C	U	U	U	C	U	U	I	U	C	I	U
Propanolol HCl (Inderal)	C	—	U	U	U	U	I	I	U	U	U	U	I	U	U	U	U	C	U	I	I	U	U	U	U
Verapamil (Isoptin)	—	C	C	U	C	C	I	I	U	U	C	C	C	C	C	C	C	C	U	U	C	I	C	C	U	C

Legend: C = Compatible; I = Incompatible; U = Unknown; S = Compatible in same syringe (use of specific reference required).

K⁺ SCALE

Give intravenously 2 mEq KCl for each 0.1 mEq below the desired serum K⁺ level.

1. Should be given in a drip, not in a bolus.
2. Should be given through a central line.
3. Except under conditions of severe hypokalemia, no more than 20 mEq of KCl in 50–100 ml D5W should be given in 1 hr.

Medication compatibility chart. C = Compatible; I = Incompatible; U = Unknown; S = Should not be mixed in same container. May be infused in same line at least 1 hr apart.

chapter 3
CARDIOVASCULAR CARE

ADVANCED CARDIAC LIFE SUPPORT ALGORITHMS

VENTRICULAR FIBRILLATION AND PULSELESS VENTRICULAR TACHYCARDIA[a]

This sequence was developed to assist in teaching how to treat a broad range of patients with ventricular fibrillation (VF) or pulseless ventricular tachycardia (VT). Some patients may require care not specified herein. This algorithm should not be construed as prohibiting such flexibility. Flow of algorithm presumes that VF is continuing. CPR indicates cardiopulmonary resuscitation.

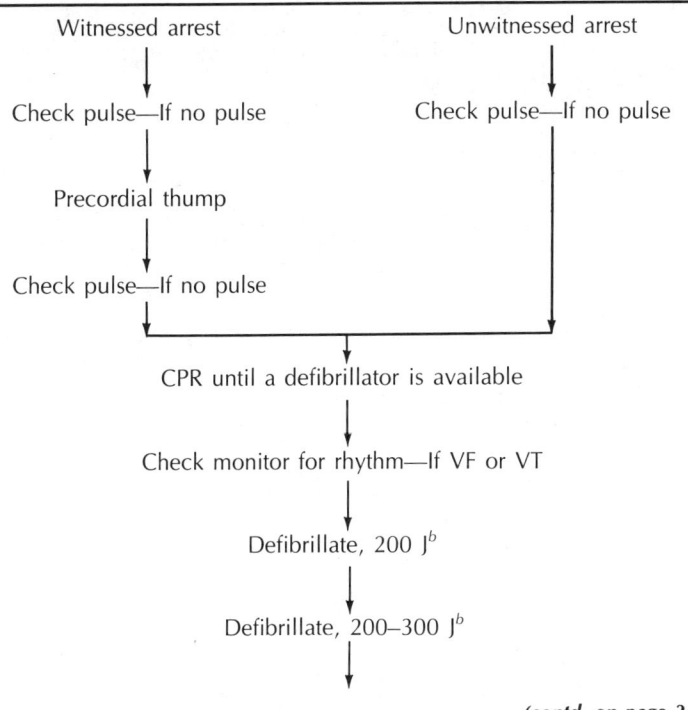

Witnessed arrest
↓
Check pulse—If no pulse
↓
Precordial thump
↓
Check pulse—If no pulse

Unwitnessed arrest
↓
Check pulse—If no pulse

↓
CPR until a defibrillator is available
↓
Check monitor for rhythm—If VF or VT
↓
Defibrillate, 200 J[b]
↓
Defibrillate, 200–300 J[b]
↓

(contd. on page 34)

Defibrillate with up to 360 J[b]

↓

CPR if no pulse

↓

Establish i.v. access

↓

Epinephrine, 1:10,000, 0.5–1.0 mg i.v. push[c]

↓

Intubate if possible[d]

↓

Defibrillate with up to 360 J[b]

↓

Lidocaine, 1 mg/kg i.v. push

↓

Defibrillate with up to 360 J[b]

↓

Bretylium, 5 mg/kg i.v. push[e]

↓

(Consider bicarbonate)[f]

↓

Defibrillate with up to 360 J[b]

↓

(contd. on page 35)

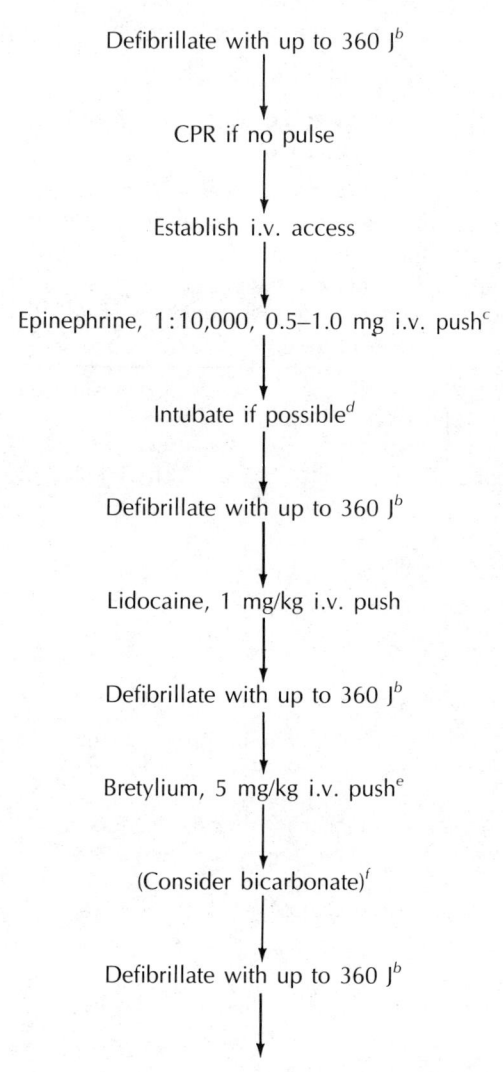

Bretylium, 10 mg/kg i.v. push[e]

↓

Defibrillate with up to 360 J[b]

↓

Repeat lidocaine or bretylium

↓

Defibrillate with up to 360 J[b]

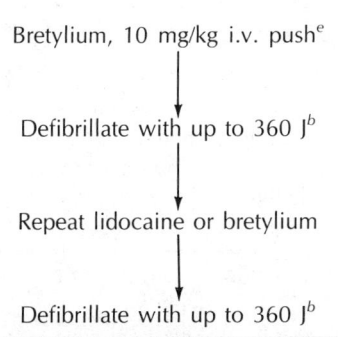

[a]Pulseless VT should be treated identically to VF.
[b]Check pulse and rhythm after each shock. If VF recurs after transiently converting (rather than persists without ever converting), use whatever energy level has previously been successful for defibrillation.
[c]Epinephrine should be repeated every 5 min.
[d]Intubation is preferable. If it can be accomplished simultaneously with other techniques, then the earlier the better. However, defibrillation and epinephrine are more important initially if the patient can be ventilated without intubation.
[e]Some may prefer repeated doses of lidocaine, which may be given in 0.5 mg/kg boluses every 8 min to a total dose of 3 mg/kg.
[f]Value of sodium bicarbonate is questionable during cardiac arrest, and it is not recommended for the routine cardiac arrest sequence. Consideration of its use in a dose of 1 mEq/kg is appropriate at this point. Half the original dose may be repeated every 10 min if it is used.
From American Heart Association. *Textbook of Advanced Cardiac Life Support.*

ASYSTOLE (CARDIAC STANDSTILL)

This sequence was developed to assist in teaching how to treat a broad range of patients with asystole. Some patients may require care not specified herein. This algorithm should not be construed to prohibit such flexibility. Flow of the algorithm presumes that asystole is continuing. VF, ventricular fibrillation; i.v., intravenous; CPR, cardiopulmonary resuscitation.

If rhythm is unclear and possibly ventricular fibrillation, defibrillate as for VF.
If asystole is present[a]

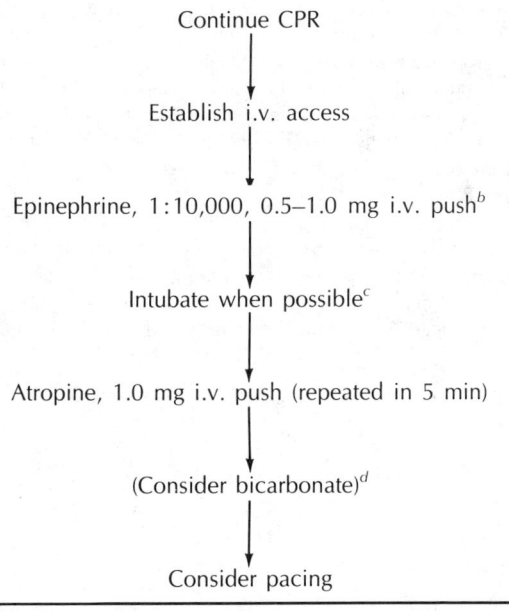

↓

Continue CPR

↓

Establish i.v. access

↓

Epinephrine, 1:10,000, 0.5–1.0 mg i.v. push[b]

↓

Intubate when possible[c]

↓

Atropine, 1.0 mg i.v. push (repeated in 5 min)

↓

(Consider bicarbonate)[d]

↓

Consider pacing

---

[a] Asystole should be confirmed in two leads.
[b] Epinephrine should be repeated every 5 min.
[c] Intubation is preferable. If it can be accomplished simultaneously with other

techniques, then the earlier the better. However, CPR and the use of epinephrine are more important initially if the patient can be ventilated without intubation. (Endotracheal epinephrine may be used.)

[d]Value of sodium bicarbonate is questionable during cardiac arrest, and it is not recommended for the routine cardiac arrest sequence. Consideration of its use in a dose of 1 mEq/kg is appropriate at this point. Half the original dose may be repeated every 10 min if it is used.

From American Heart Association. *Textbook of Advanced Cardiac Life Support.*

ELECTROMECHANICAL DISSOCIATION

This sequence was developed to assist in teaching how to treat a broad range of patients with electromechanical dissociation. Some patients may require care not specified herein. This algorithm should not be construed to prohibit such flexibility. Flow of the algorithm presumes that electromechanical dissociation is continuing. CPR, cardiopulmonary resuscitation; i.v., intravenous.

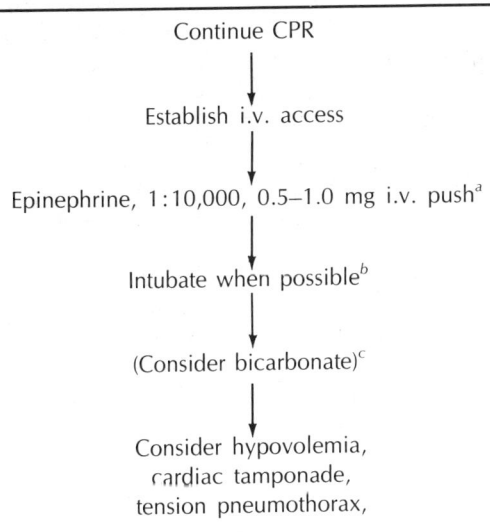

Continue CPR
↓
Establish i.v. access
↓
Epinephrine, 1:10,000, 0.5–1.0 mg i.v. push[a]
↓
Intubate when possible[b]
↓
(Consider bicarbonate)[c]
↓
Consider hypovolemia,
cardiac tamponade,
tension pneumothorax,

(contd. on page 38)

hypoxemia,
acidosis,
pulmonary embolism

---

[a]Epinephrine should be repeated every 5 min.

[b]Intubation is preferable. If it can be accomplished simultaneously with other techniques, then the earlier the better. However, epinephrine is more important initially if the patient can be ventilated without intubation. (Endotracheal epinephrine may be used.)

[c]Value of sodium bicarbonate is questionable during cardiac arrest, and it is not recommended for the routine cardiac arrest sequence. Consideration of its use in a dose of 1 mEq/kg is appropriate at this point. Half the original dose may be repeated every 10 min if it is used.

From American Heart Association. *Textbook of Advanced Cardiac Life Support.*

SUSTAINED VENTRICULAR TACHYCARDIA

This sequence was developed to assist in teaching how to treat a broad range of patients with sustained VT. Some patients may require care not specified herein. This algorithm should not be construed to prohibit such flexibility. Flow of the algorithm presumes that VT is continuing. VF, ventricular fibrillation; i.v., intravenous.

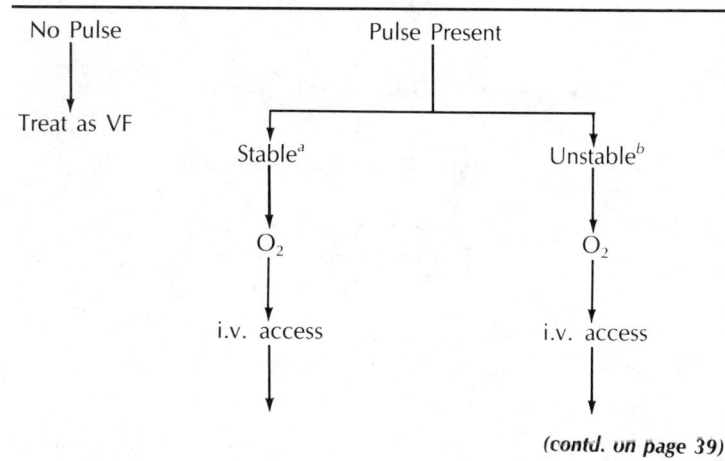

No Pulse → Treat as VF

Pulse Present
- Stable[a] → O_2 → i.v. access
- Unstable[b] → O_2 → i.v. access

(contd. on page 39)

Lidocaine, 0.5 mg/kg every 8 min until VT resolves, or up to 3 mg/kg	(Consider sedation)[c]
↓	↓
Procainamide, 20 mg/min until VT resolves or up to 1000 mg	Cardiovert 50 J[d,e]
	↓
	Cardiovert 100 J[d]
↓	↓
	Cardiovert 200 J[d]
Cardiovert as in unstable patients[c]	↓
	Cardiovert with up to 360 J[d]
	↓
	If recurrent, add lidocaine and cardiovert again starting at energy level previously successful, then procainamide or bretylium[f]

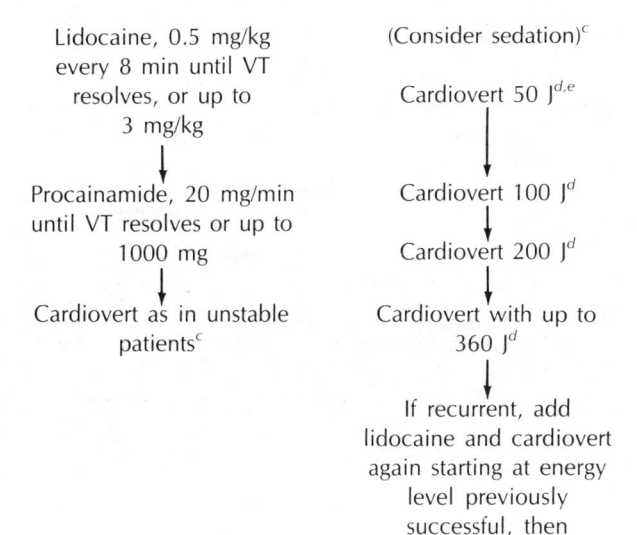

---

[a] If a patient becomes unstable (see footnote *b* for definition) at any time, move to "Unstable" arm of the algorithm.

[b] Unstable indicates symptoms (e.g., chest pain or dyspnea), hypotension (systolic blood pressure <90 mm Hg), congestive heart failure, ischemia, or infarction.

[c] Sedation should be considered for all patients, including those defined in footnote *b* as unstable (e.g., hypotensive, in pulmonary edema, or unconscious).

[d] If hypotension, pulmonary edema, or unconsciousness is present, unsynchronized cardioversion should be done to avoid delay associated with synchronization.

[e] In the absence of hypotension, pulmonary edema, or unconsciousness, a precordial thump may be employed prior to cardioversion.

[f] Once VT has been resolved, begin i.v. infusion of antiarrhythmic agent that has aided resolution of VT. If hypotension, pulmonary edema, or unconsciousness is present, use lidocaine if cardioversion alone is unsuccessful, followed by bretylium. In all other patients, recommended order of therapy is lidocaine, procainamide, and then bretylium.

Reproduced with permission.

From American Heart Association. *Textbook of Advanced Cardiac Life Support.*

BRADYCARDIA

This sequence was developed to assist in teaching how to treat a broad range of patients with bradycardia. Some patients may require care not specified herein. This algorithm should not be construed to prohibit such flexibility. A-V, atrioventricular.

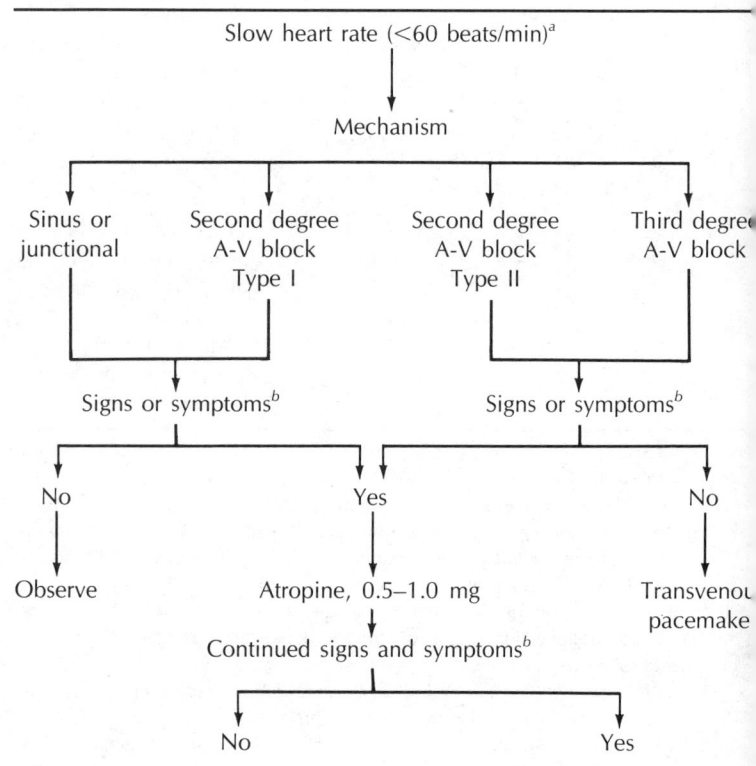

```
                    Slow heart rate (<60 beats/min)ᵃ
                                  │
                                  ▼
                             Mechanism
         ┌────────────────┬──────────────────┬────────────────┐
         ▼                ▼                  ▼                ▼
      Sinus or      Second degree      Second degree     Third degree
      junctional      A-V block          A-V block        A-V block
                       Type I             Type II
         └────────────────┘                  └────────────────┘
                  ▼                                   ▼
          Signs or symptomsᵇ                 Signs or symptomsᵇ
           ┌──────┴──────┐                    ┌──────┴──────┐
           ▼             ▼                    ▼             ▼
          No            Yes                  Yes            No
           ▼             ▼                                  ▼
        Observe    Atropine, 0.5–1.0 mg                Transvenous
                          ▼                             pacemaker
                Continued signs and symptomsᵇ
                    ┌─────┴─────┐
                    ▼           ▼
                   No          Yes
```

(contd. on page 41)

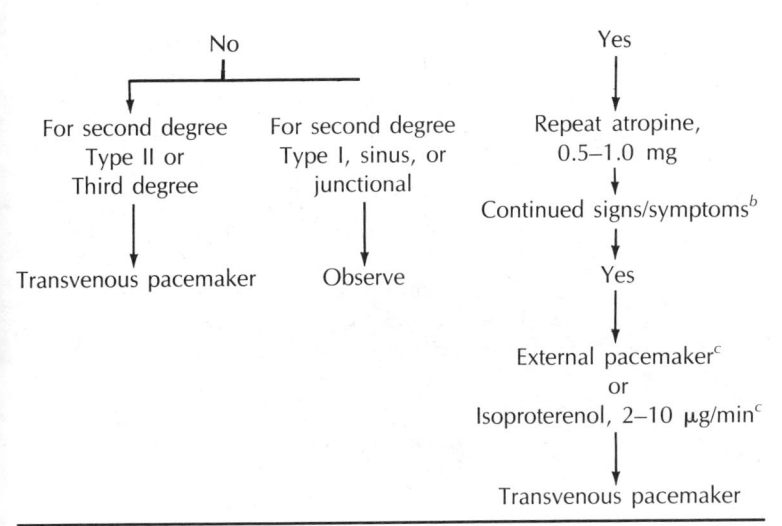

```
            No                                    Yes
            |                                      |
    ┌───────┴───────┐                              ▼
    ▼               ▼                     Repeat atropine,
For second degree   For second degree        0.5–1.0 mg
Type II or          Type I, sinus, or             |
Third degree        junctional                    ▼
    |                   |                 Continued signs/symptoms[b]
    ▼                   ▼                         |
Transvenous pacemaker   Observe                   ▼
                                                 Yes
                                                  |
                                                  ▼
                                         External pacemaker[c]
                                                  or
                                       Isoproterenol, 2–10 µg/min[c]
                                                  |
                                                  ▼
                                         Transvenous pacemaker
```

[a] A solitary chest thump or cough may stimulate cardiac electrical activity and result in improved cardiac output and may be used at this point.
[b] Hypotension (blood pressure <90 mm Hg), premature ventricular contractions, altered mental status or symptoms (e.g., chest pain or dyspnea), ischemia, or infarction.
[c] Temporizing therapy.
From American Heart Association. *Textbook of Advanced Cardiac Life Support.*

VENTRICULAR ECTOPY: ACUTE SUPPRESSIVE THERAPY

This sequence was developed to assist in teaching how to treat a broad range of patients with ventricular ectopy. Some patients may require care not specified herein. This algorithm should not be construed to prohibit such flexibility.

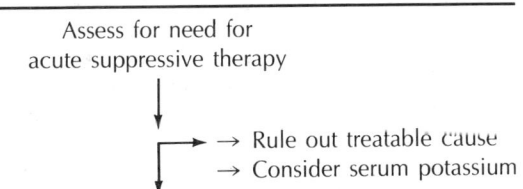

```
              Assess for need for
           acute suppressive therapy
                      |
                      ▼
                      ┌─→  Rule out treatable cause
                      │    Consider serum potassium
                      ▼
```

→ Consider digitalis level
→ Consider bradycardia
→ Consider drugs

↓

Lidocaine, 1 mg/kg

↓

If not suppressed,
repeat lidocaine, 0.5 mg/kg every 2–5 min,
until no ectopy, or up to 3 mg/kg given

↓

If not suppressed,
procainamide 20 mg/min
until no ectopy, or up to 1000 mg given

↓

If not suppressed,
and not contraindicated,
bretylium, 5–10 mg/kg over 8–10 min

↓

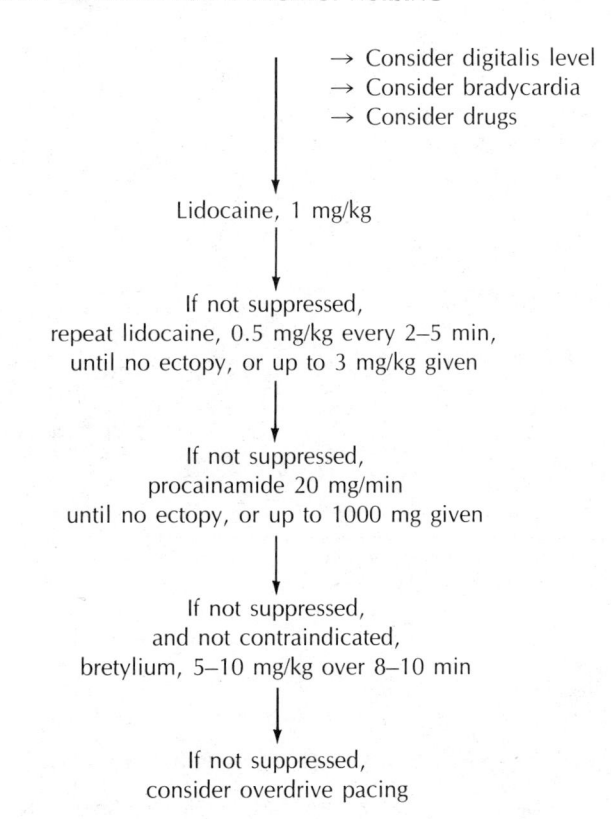

If not suppressed,
consider overdrive pacing

Once ectopy resolved, maintain as follows:
  After lidocaine, 1 mg/kg . . . lidocaine drip, 2 mg/min
  After lidocaine, 1–2 mg/kg . . . lidocaine drip, 3 mg/min
  After lidocaine, 2–3 mg/kg . . . lidocaine drip, 4 mg/min
  After procainamide . . . procainamide drip, 1–4 mg/min (check blood level)
  After bretylium . . . bretylium drip, 2 mg/min

From American Heart Association. *Textbook of Advanced Cardiac Life Support.*

PAROXYSMAL SUPRAVENTRICULAR TACHYCARDIA (PSVT)

This sequence was developed to assist in teaching how to treat a broad range of patients with sustained PSVT. Some patients may require care not specified herein. This algorithm should not be construed to prohibit such flexibility. Flow of algorithm presumes PSVT is continuing.

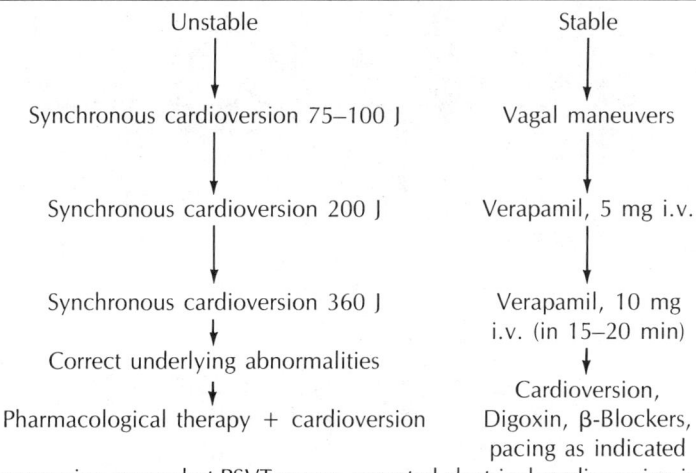

Unstable	Stable
↓	↓
Synchronous cardioversion 75–100 J	Vagal maneuvers
↓	↓
Synchronous cardioversion 200 J	Verapamil, 5 mg i.v.
↓	↓
Synchronous cardioversion 360 J	Verapamil, 10 mg i.v. (in 15–20 min)
↓	↓
Correct underlying abnormalities	Cardioversion, Digoxin, β-Blockers, pacing as indicated
↓	
Pharmacological therapy + cardioversion	

If conversion occurs but PSVT recurs, repeated electrical cardioversion is *not* indicated. Sedation should be used as time permits.

From American Heart Association. *Textbook of Advanced Cardiac Life Support.*

LEAD PLACEMENT

Lead I placement.

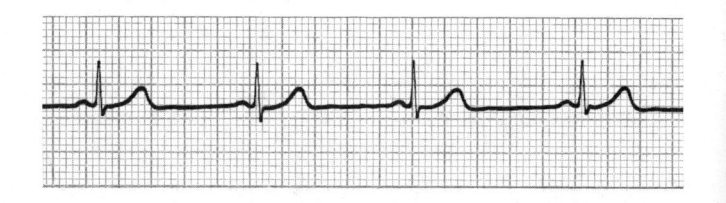

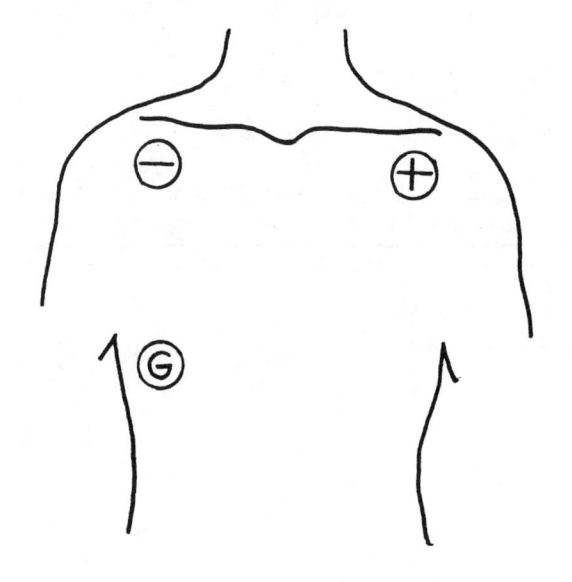

chapter 3: **CARDIOVASCULAR CARE** 45

Lead II placement.

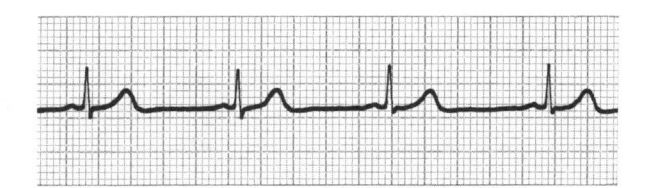

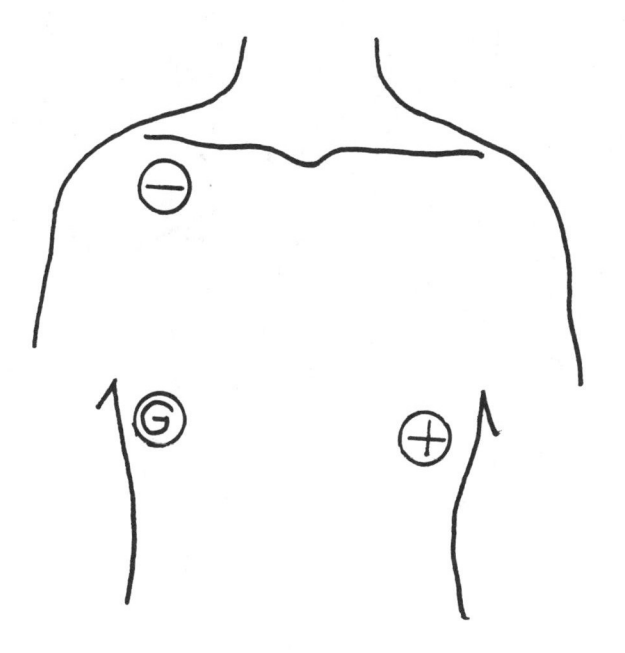

46　READY REFERENCE FOR EMERGENCY NURSING

Lead III placement.

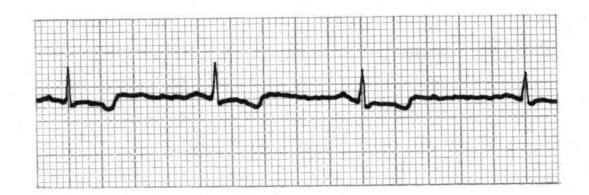

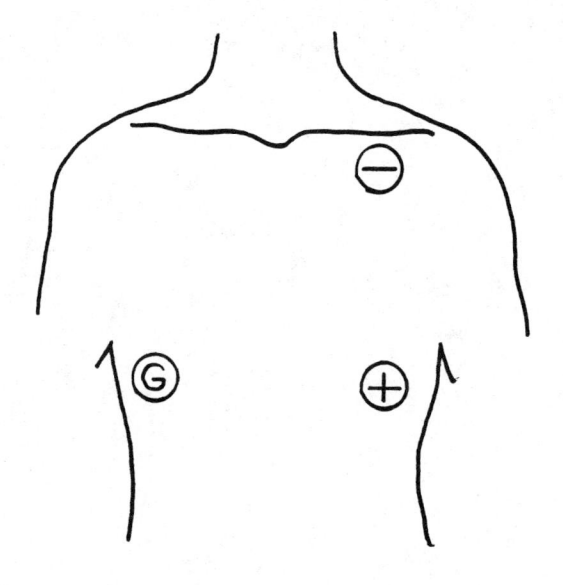

chapter 3: **CARDIOVASCULAR CARE** 47

MCL1 placement.

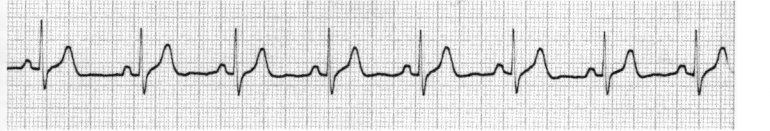

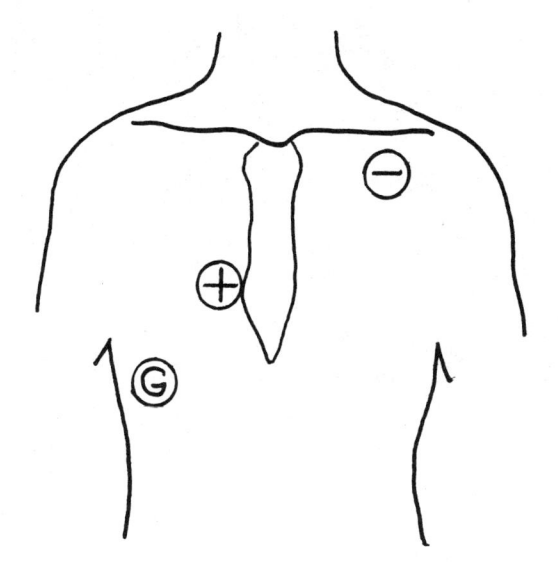

48 READY REFERENCE FOR EMERGENCY NURSING

PRECORDIAL (V) LEAD PLACEMENT

V_1 and V_2 are on either side of the sternum, at the fourth intercostal space.
V_4 is at the midclavicular line, fifth intercostal space.
V_3 is halfway between V_2 and V_4.
V_5 is at the fifth intercostal space, anterior axillary line.
V_6 is at the fifth intercostal space, midaxillary line.

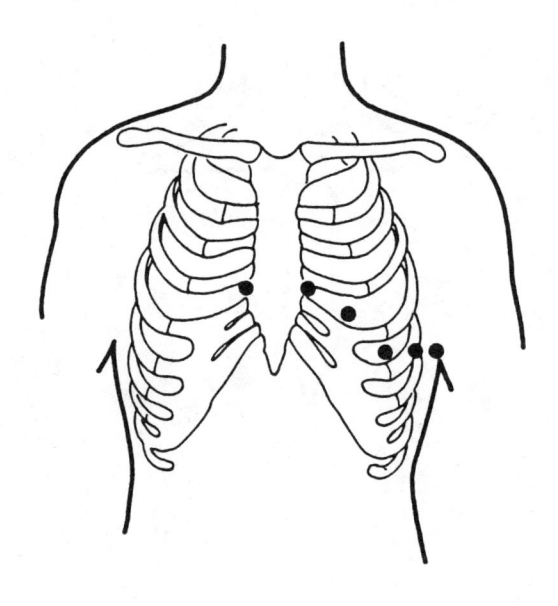

chapter **3**: CARDIOVASCULAR CARE   49

NORMAL ELECTROCARDIOGRAM INTERVALS AND RATE DETERMINATION

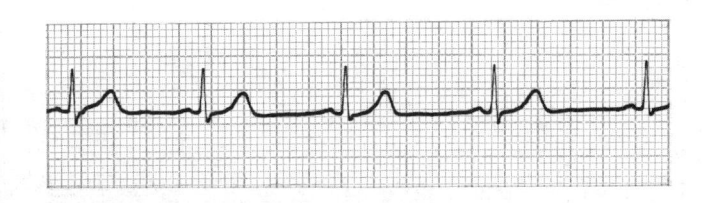

From one dark line to the next: 0.20 sec
From one light line to the next: 0.04 sec
The single vertical lines above the grid can be every second or every 3 sec.
Normal P-R interval: 0.12–0.20 sec
Normal QRS interval: less than 0.12 sec
Normal Q-T interval: less than 1/2 the preceding R-R interval
Rate determination:
  If the ryhthm is irregular, count the number of R waves during a 6-second interval and multiply by 10 to get beats per minute.
  If the rhythm is regular, the above technique can be used, or count the number of dark large squares between two R waves and divide that number into 300.
  For very fast rhythms, count the number of small light squares between the R waves and divide that number into 1500.
  Atrial rates can be determined by substituting P waves for R waves.

12-LEAD ECG INTERPRETATION

Myocardial ischemia: Symmetrically inverted T wave in leads that look directly at ischemic area.

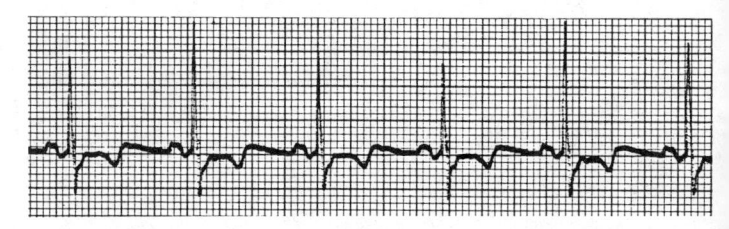

Acute injury: Elevated S-T segment in leads that look directly at injured area.

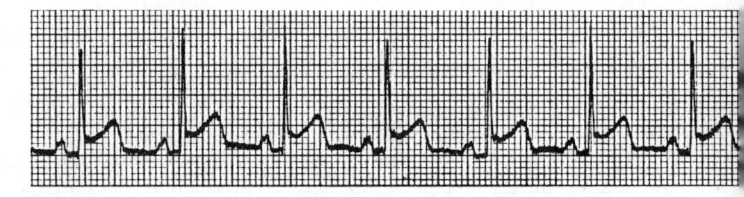

Myocardial infarction: Significant Q waves: width is greater than 0.03 sec, or depth is greater than 25% of the R wave.

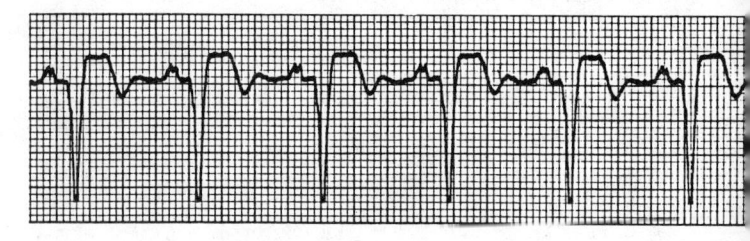

chapter 3: CARDIOVASCULAR CARE 51

Digitalis effect: Asymmetrically depressed S-T segment in leads where QRS is positive. Short Q-T interval.

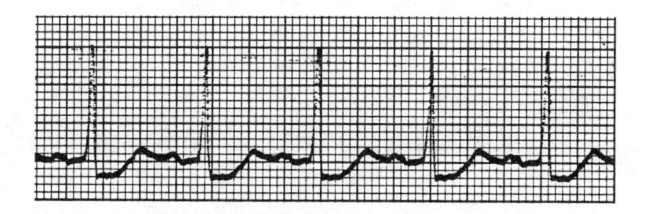

Strain pattern: Depressed S-T Segment and inverted T wave.

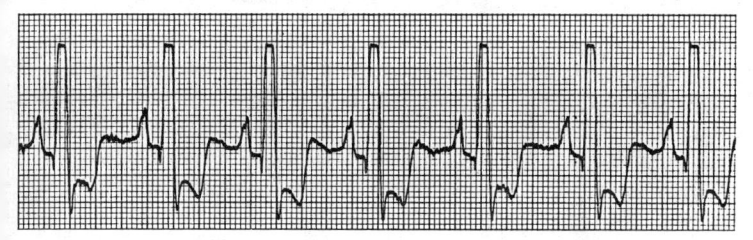

Anterior myocardial infarction: Significant Q waves in leads V_2 through V_4.

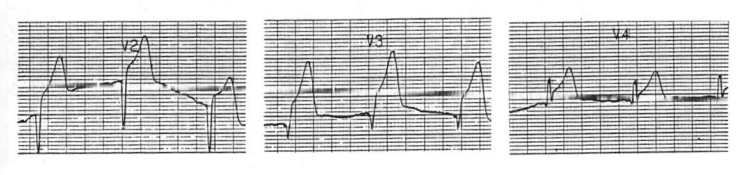

52 READY REFERENCE FOR EMERGENCY NURSING

Anteroseptal myocardial infarction: Significant Q waves in leads V_1 through V_3.

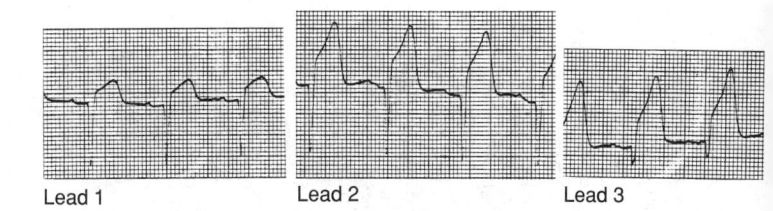

Lead 1   Lead 2   Lead 3

Anterolateral myocardial infarction: Significant Q waves in leads I, aV_L and V_4 through V_6.

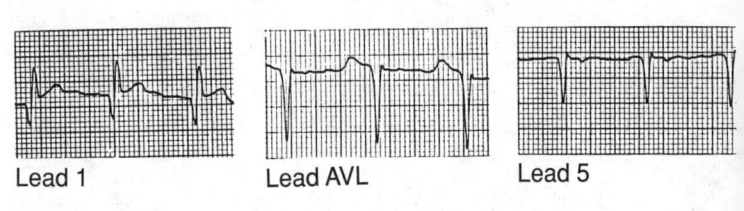

Lead 1   Lead AVL   Lead 5

Inferior myocardial infarction: Significant Q waves in leads II, III, aV_F.

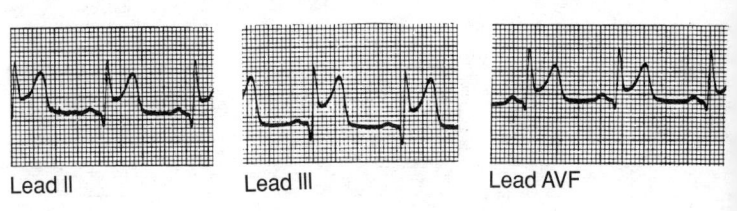

Lead II   Lead III   Lead AVF

chapter 3: **CARDIOVASCULAR CARE** 53

Posterior myocardial infarction: Tall R waves in V_1 through V_3. S-T depression in V_1 through V_3. T wave upright.

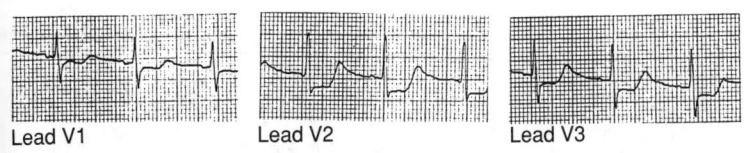

Lead V1   Lead V2   Lead V3

Subendocardial myocardial infarction: No significant Q waves. Symmetrical T wave inversion. Depressed S-T segment. Some loss of R waves.

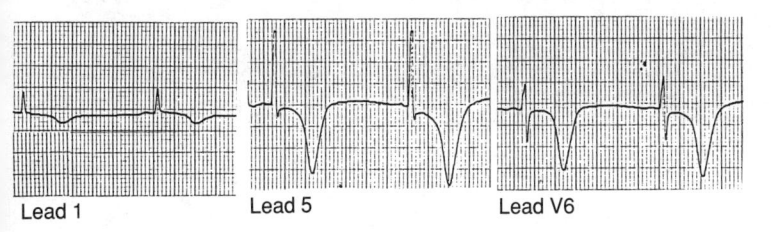

Lead 1   Lead 5   Lead V6

INTRAVASCULAR PRESSURES

Central venous pressure (CVP): 6–8 cm H_2O or 2–6 mm Hg
Mean arterial pressure (MAP): 70–105 mm Hg

$$MAP = \frac{Pulse\ Pressure}{3} + Diastolic\ Pressure$$

Right atrial (RA) pressure: 2–6 mm Hg
Right ventricular (RV) pressure: $25/2$–$25/6$ mm Hg
Pulmonary artery (PA) pressure: $25/8$–$25/12$ mm Hg
Pulmonary artery wedge (PAW) pressure: 8–12 mm Hg
Coronary perfusion pressure (CPP): 60–70 mm Hg

$$CPP = Diastolic\ blood\ pressure - PAW$$

Pulmonary artery catheter positions and corresponding waveforms. Courtesy of Baxter Healthcare Corporation.

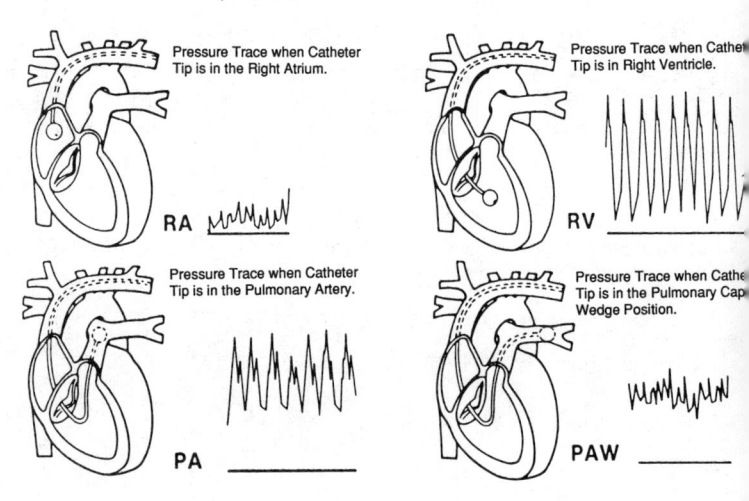

Pressure Trace when Catheter Tip is in the Right Atrium.

RA

Pressure Trace when Catheter Tip is in Right Ventricle.

RV

Pressure Trace when Catheter Tip is in the Pulmonary Artery.

PA

Pressure Trace when Catheter Tip is in the Pulmonary Capillary Wedge Position.

PAW

POSTURAL (ORTHOSTATIC) BLOOD PRESSURE AND PULSE

Take the blood pressure and pulse while the patient is supine. Then sit the patient up and dangle his or her legs over the side of the stretcher. Immediately measure pulse and blood pressure again. Any one of three changes indicates significant volume loss:

1. A rise in the pulse rate of 20 beats per minute or more
2. A drop in blood pressure of 20 mm Hg or more
3. Symptoms of dizziness, light-headedness, weakness

Pulsus Paradoxus:

In significant pulsus paradoxus, the systolic blood pressure drops at least 10 mm Hg during inspiration.

While patient is breathing normally, inflate blood pressure cuff, then deflate it slowly until the first sound is heard. Watch the patient's respirations to see if the sound fades away during inspiration. Continue to deflate the cuff until all sounds are heard. The difference between the pressure when sounds were first heard and when all the sounds were heard is the paradox.

Pulsus paradoxus may indicate severe lung disease, severe heart failure, pericardial tamponade, or pericarditis.

Pulsus Alternans:

In pulsus alternans, the heart beats regularly, but the amount of systolic blood pressure alternates with each beat.

Inflate the blood pressure cuff, then slowly deflate it. Initially, only alternate beats will be heard, then softer sounds will emerge as the cuff is deflated, or suddenly the number of beats will double. Pulsus alternans may be indicative of left ventricular failure.

chapter 4

PULMONARY CARE

chapter **4: PULMONARY CARE** 59

OXYGEN DELIVERY SYSTEMS

Device	Oxygen Delivery	Comments
Nasal cannula	22–30%	Maximum flow advised: 6 liters/min.
Partial rebreather mask	Up to 60%	Air ports on sides of mask are open. Provide enough oxygen flow rate to ensure that bag is full, deflating slightly during inspiration. Minimal flow rate: 5 liters/min.
Nonrebreather mask	Up to 90%	Air ports on sides of mask are sealed during inspiration. Provide enough oxygen flow rate to ensure that bag is full, deflating slightly during inspiration. Minimal flow rate: 5 liters/min.
Venturi mask	24–50%	Green adjuster, green settings; white adjuster, white settings. Flow rate as indicated on settings.
Bag-valve-mask	Up to 100%	Must have a reservoir. Flow rate: 15 liters/min.

ABBREVIATIONS AND TERMS

Respiratory Physiology

(General)	(Gas Phase)	(Blood Phase)
P—Pressure	A—Alveolar	a—Arterial
$\bar{X}$—A mean value	D—Dead space	c—Capillary
$\dot{X}$—A time derivative	E—Expired	$\dot{Q}$—Blood flow
	F—Fractional	Q—Blood volume

concentration of a gas
I —Inspired
T —Tidal
V —Gas volume
v —Venous
$\bar{v}$ —Mixed venous

Measurements of Ventilation
CC—Closing capacity
CV—Closing volume
FRC—Functional residual capacity
TV (or VT)—Tidal volume
VA—Alveolar ventilation
VC—Vital capacity
VD—Dead-space ventilation
VD/VT—Dead-space/Tidal volume ratio
$\dot{V}E$—Minute expired volume
$\dot{V}I$—Minute inspired volume

Measurement of Mechanics of Breathing
C—Compliance
PAW—Airway pressure
PIP—Peak inspiratory pressure
R—Resistance
W—Work of breathing

Miscellaneous
$C(a-v)O_2$ —Arteriovenous oxygen content difference
CMV —Controlled mechanical ventilation
CPAP —Continuous positive airway pressure = EPAP + IPAP
CPPB —Continuous positive pressure breathing
CPPV —Continuous positive pressure ventilation
EPAP —Expiratory positive airway pressure
IAV —Intermittent assisted ventilation
IDV —Intermittent demand ventilation
IMV —Intermittent mandatory ventilation
IPAP —Inspiratory positive airway pressure
PEEP —Positive end-expiratory pressure
$P(A-a)O_2$ —Alveolar-arterial oxygen pressure difference
Qsp —Physiologic shunt flow (total venous admixture); often expressed as percent of cardiac output

SIMV —Synchronized intermittent mandatory ventilation
SPEEP —Spontaneous positive end-expiratory pressure

INITIAL VENTILATOR SETTINGS

Tidal volume: 10 ml/kg of body weight
Rate: 15 breaths per minute
FiO_2: Depends on condition of patient. Usually between 60 and 80%. Test arterial blood gases 30 min after initiation of ventilator.

Oxyhemoglobin dissociation curve.

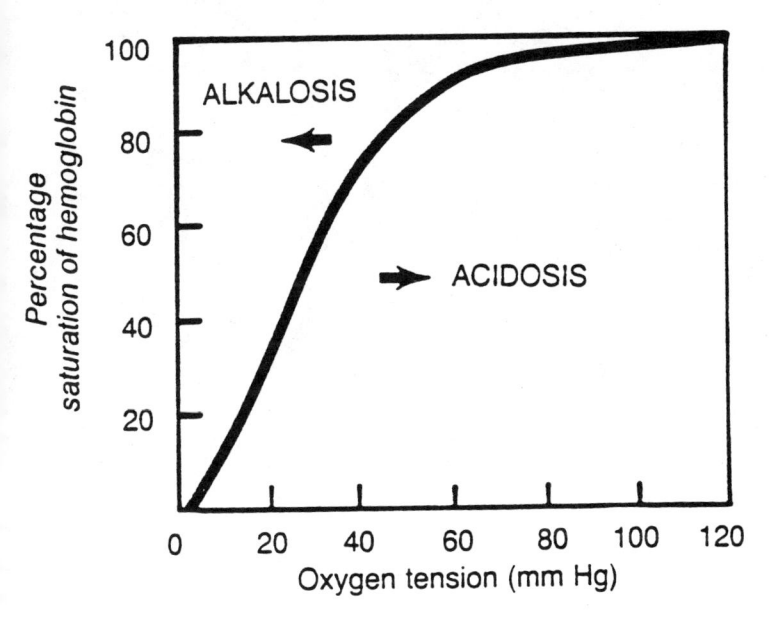

chapter 5

NEUROLOGIC CARE

chapter **5: NEUROLOGICAL CARE** 65

GLASGOW COMA SCALE

Score in each category, then total the scores. Highest score is 15; lowest score is 3.

Finding	Score
Eye opening	
Spontaneous	4
To voice	3
To pain	2
None	1
Best verbal response	
Oriented	5
Confused	4
Inappropriate words	3
Incomprehensible words	2
None	1
Best motor response	
Obeys commands	6
Localizes to pain	5
Withdraws from pain	4
Flexion to pain (decorticate posturing)	3
Extension to pain (decerebrate posturing)	2
None	1
Total	___

INTRACRANIAL PRESSURE

Normal Intracranial Pressure (ICP) is 0 to 15 mm Hg.
Monitor wave patterns
    "A" or plateau waves — increases in ICP to 50 to 100 mm Hg for 5 to 20 min. These occur with a mean ICP of 20 mm Hg and are considered to be an indication of ICP decompensation.

"B" waves—sharp, rhythmic oscillation occurring every ½ to 2 min; range in amplitude, from 0 to 50 mm Hg. They relate to changes in respiration patterns.

"C" waves—usually occur with a frequency of 4 to 8 per min and an amplitude of from 0 to 20 mm Hg. They correlate with normal fluctuations in arterial pressure.

chapter 5: **NEUROLOGICAL CARE** 67

Dermatome chart.

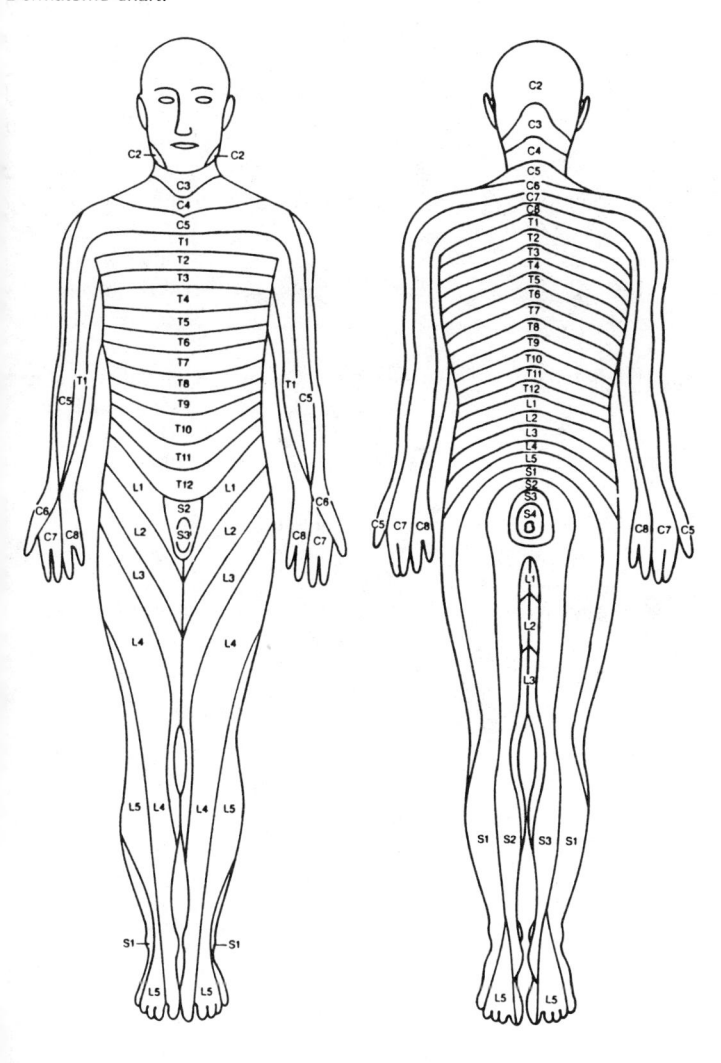

CRANIAL NERVE TESTING

Nerve		Function	Test
I	Olfactory	Smell	Identify coffee grounds with eyes closed
II	Optic	Vision	Visual acuities
III	Oculomotor	Eye movement	Follow finger inward and upward
IV	Trochlear	Eye movement	Follow finger downward and outward
V	Trigeminal	Chewing, facial sensations	Corneal reflex, feel light touch on cheek
VI	Abducens	Eye movement	Follow finger to side
VII	Facial	Facial expressions, taste, salivation, tearing	Symmetry of smile, taste salt
VIII	Acoustic	Hearing, equilibrium	Hear whispered words
IX	Glossopharyngeal	Salivation, swallowing, taste	Taste sweet
X	Vagus	Swallowing, heart rate, peristalsis, talk	Gag reflex, talk is hoarse
XI	Accessory	Shoulder, neck movement	Shrug shoulders, rotate head
XII	Hypoglossal	Tongue movement	Protrude tongue

chapter 5: **NEUROLOGICAL CARE** 69

Pupil size chart.

MILLIMETERS

- 1.0 •
- 1.5 •
- 2.0 •
- 2.5 •
- 3.0 •
- 3.5 •
- 4.0 •
- 4.5 •
- 5.0 •
- 5.5 •
- 6.0 •
- 6.5 •
- 7.0 •

Normal size of adult pupil: 2.9 to 6.5 mm.

chapter 6

ORTHOPAEDIC CARE

APPLICATION OF AN ORTHOPAEDIC CASTING LABORATORY (OCL) SPLINT

1. Properly dress wounds before applying splint, if applicable.
2. Apply foam side of splint next to patient.
3. Do not wrap too tightly—allow for edema.
4. Patient should not bear weight on splints.
5. Flare back exposed edges.

POSTERIOR SPLINT OF ANKLE (DARTED). Material Width: 6 inches, adult; 4–5 inches, child. Template: None. (Courtesy of Orthopedic Casting Laboratory, Inc.)

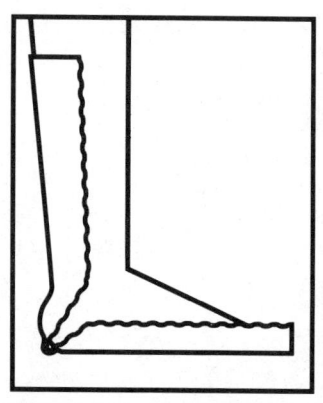

STEP 1: Measure length from toes to desired height below knee. Cut this length of splint roll.

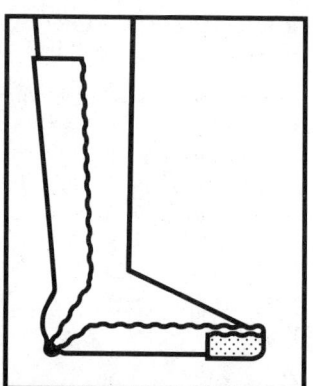

STEP 2: After general preparation, apply foam side of splint next to patient. Fold or flare back plaster at toes.

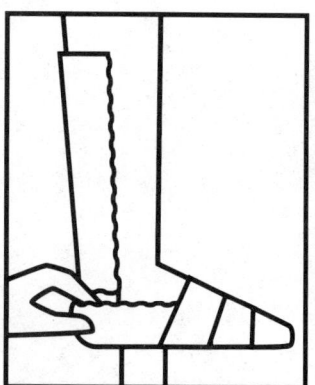

STEP 3: Form a smooth dart (tuck) in fold at heel area.

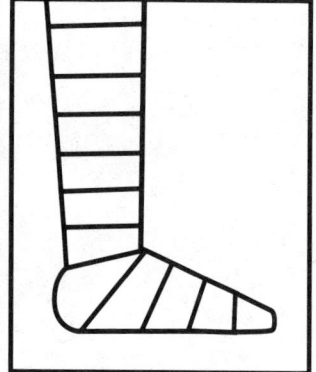

STEP 4: Secure with elastic bandage, flare back plaster below knee and position.

POSTERIOR SPLINT OF ANKLE (REINFORCED). Material Width: 6 inches, adult; 4–5 inches, child. Template: None. (Courtesy of Orthopedic Casting Laboratory, Inc.)

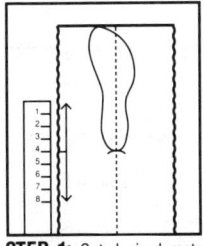

STEP 1: Cut desired material length. After general preparation, measure length of foot from heel to toes and make indent. Measure 4'' to either side of indent and mark.

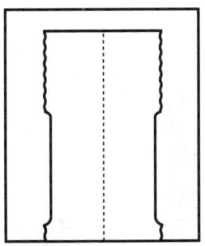

STEP 2: Trim away sewn edges between points. DO NOT CUT INTO PLASTER.

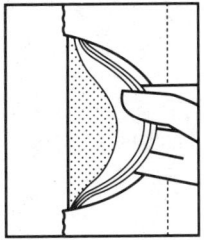

STEP 3: Lift flannel. Fold plaster layers back to center seam.

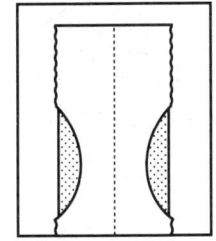

STEP 4: Tuck flannel in under plaster and smooth.

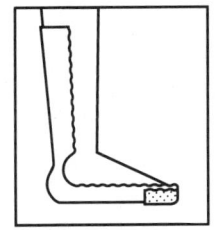

STEP 5: Apply foam side of splint next to patient. Fold or flare back plaster at toes.

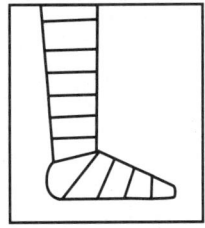

STEP 6: Secure with elastic bandage, flare back plaster below knee and position.

76 READY REFERENCE FOR EMERGENCY NURSING

STIRRUP ANKLE. Material Width: 4, 5, or 6 inches, depending on patient's size. Template: None. (Courtesy of Orthopedic Casting Laboratory, Inc.)

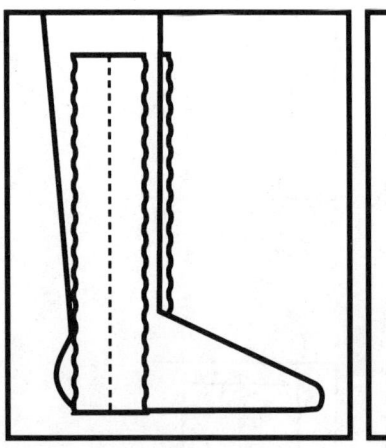

STEP 1: After general preparation, apply foam side of splint next to patient, extending splint to mid-calf.

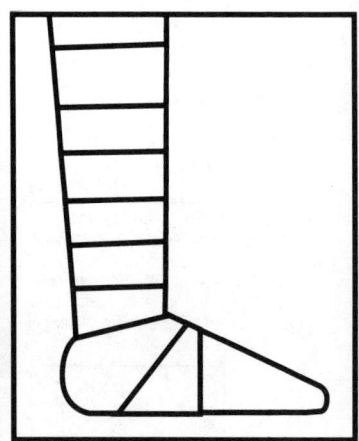

STEP 2: Secure with elastic bandage and position.

COMMON FOREARM AND HAND SPLINTS. Material Width: 3, 4, or 5 inches, adult; 2, 3, or 4 inches, child. Template: None. (Courtesy of Orthopedic Casting Laboratory, Inc.)

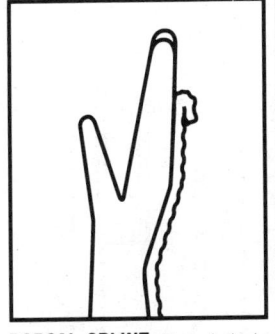

DORSAL SPLINT: Place desired length on dorsal area. Secure with elastic bandage and position.

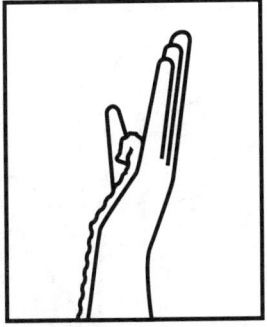

VOLAR COCK-UP: Place desired length on volar area. Secure with elastic bandage and position.

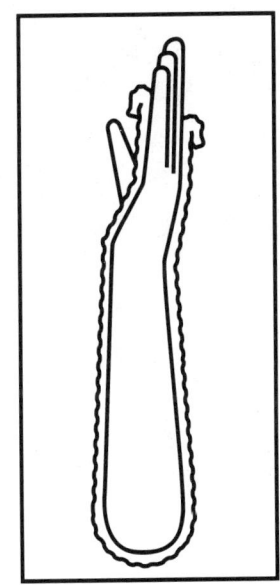

GUTTER SPLINT: Form "gutter" with desired length. Pad between fingers "buddied" together. Secure with elastic bandage and position.

SUGAR TONG: Extend length of splint roll around elbow, incorporating desired part of hand. Secure with elastic bandage and position.

BOXER SPLINT. Material Width: 3 inches, child; 4 inches, adolescent; 6 inches, adult. Template: Boxer, modified boxer with notch. Note: This splint should be made using only OCL brand splint roll. (Courtesy of Orthopedic Casting Laboratory, Inc.)

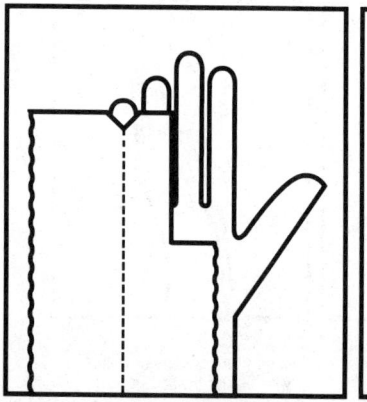

STEP 1: After general splint preparation, make appropriate cuts. Position splint on hand. If notch is used, tip of 5th finger should be exposed.

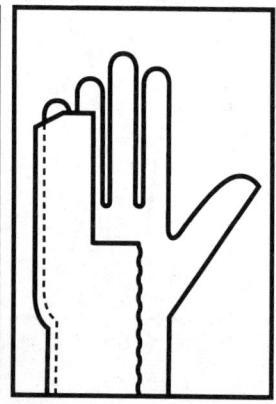

STEP 2: Fold splint to form desired gutter, place flap in palm of hand.

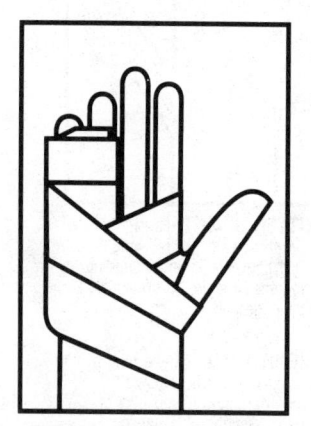

STEP 3: Pad between "buddied" fingers. Secure with elastic bandage and position.

CARPAL SPLINT. Material Width: 3 inches, child; 4 inches, adolescent; 6 inches, adult. Template: Carpal. Note: This splint should be made using only OCL brand splint roll. (Courtesy of Orthopedic Casting Laboratory, Inc.)

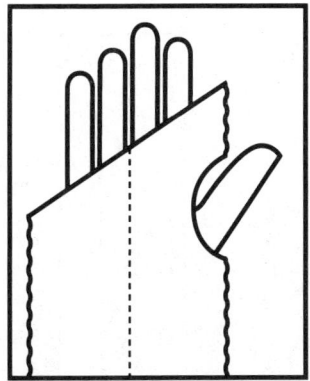

STEP 1: After general splint preparation, make appropriate cuts. Place splint, with semi-circle cut-out toward thumb, on the patient.

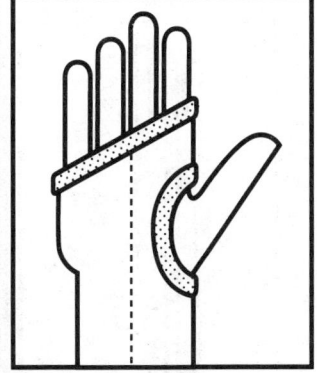

STEP 2: Flare plaster back to desired area in palm of hand and around thumb.

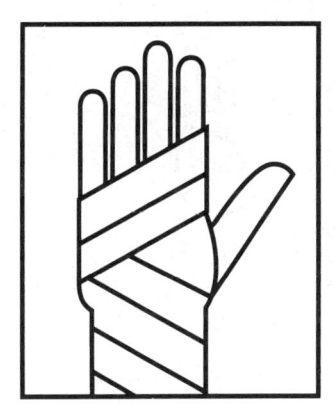

STEP 3: Secure with elastic bandage and position.

REVERSE SUGAR TONG. Material Width: 3 inches, small to medium bone structure; 4 inches, medium to large bone structure. Template: None. Note: This splint should be made using only OCL brand splint roll. (Courtesy of Orthopedic Casting Laboratory, Inc.)

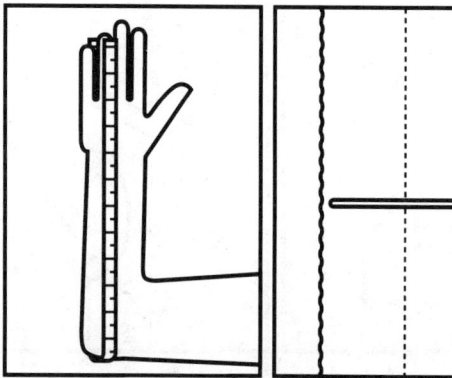

STEP 1: Measure from finger tips around elbow using unaffected arm. Cut this length of splint roll.

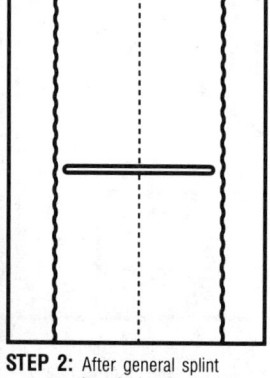

STEP 2: After general splint preparation, fold splint in half, lengthwise, making indent at midpoint. LEAVING SIDE SEAMS INTACT, make slit through splint at midpoint.

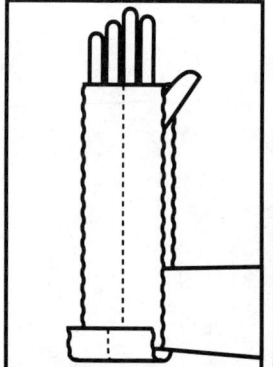

STEP 3: Slip hand through slit, positioning splint on desired area of the hand.

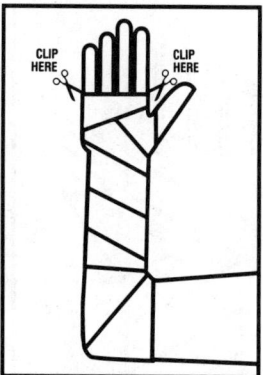

STEP 4: Begin wrapping at wrist moving toward elbow. Tuck one end under, other end over at elbow. After positioning, clip side seam in hand area to prevent constriction.

TEARDROP SPLINT. Material Width: 3 inches, child; 4 inches, adolescent; 6 inches, adult. Template: Teardrop—dorsal or volar cutout. Note: This splint should be made using only OCL brand splint roll. (Courtesy of Orthopedic Casting Laboratory, Inc.)

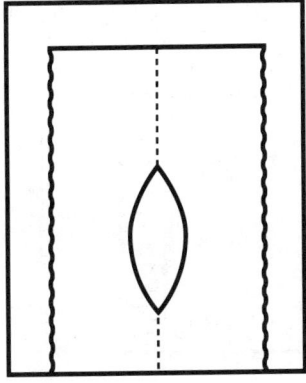

STEP 1: After general splint preparation, cut thumb hole and cut dorsal or volar flap (if desired).

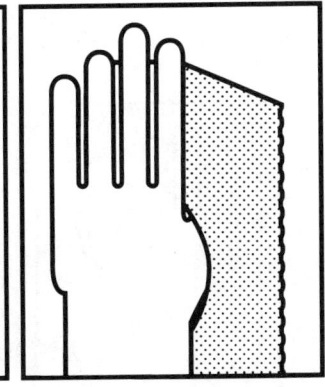

STEP 2: Place thumb through opening and flare back plaster edges. Drape splint around wrist.

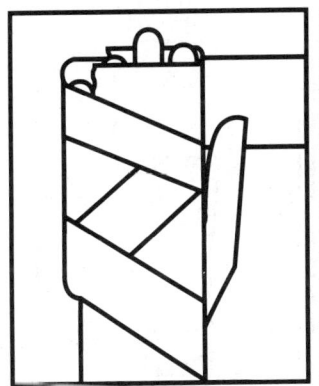

STEP 3: Secure with elastic bandage and position.

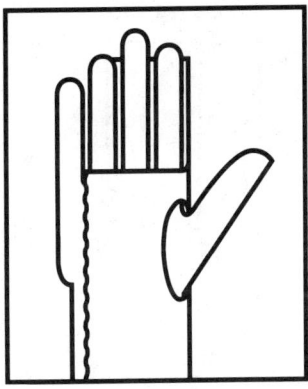

OPTIONAL CUT-OUTS: Volar or dorsal cut-outs may be used as needed.

82 READY REFERENCE FOR EMERGENCY NURSING

THUMB SPICA. Material Width: 3 inches, child; 4 inches, adolescent; 6 inches, adult. Template: Thumb spica. Note: This splint should be made using only OCL brand splint roll. (Courtesy of Orthopedic Casting Laboratory, Inc.)

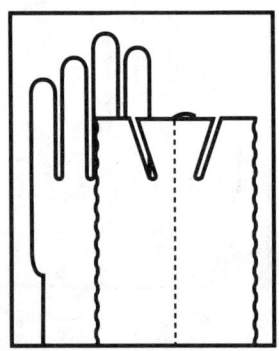

STEP 1: After general splint preparation, cut "wedge" area. Flare plaster toward flannel on flaps. Place "wedge" area around thumb, draping splint around wrist.

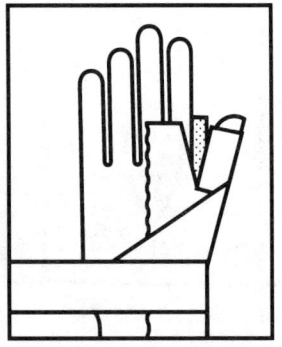

STEP 2: Secure splint at wrist or thumb.

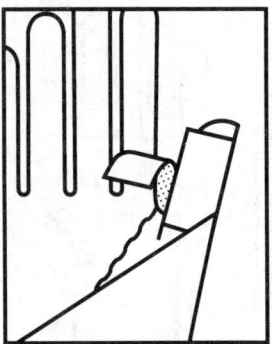

STEP 3: Tuck flap, from palmar side, around base of thumb making sure padding is in the web space. Overlap with the other flap.

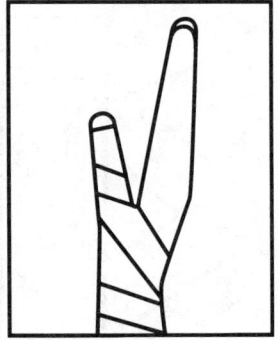

STEP 4: Finish securing with elastic bandage and position.

COMPARTMENT PRESSURE MEASUREMENT

Normal compartment pressure is less than 15 mm Hg. More than 30 mm Hg usually indicates a need for fasciotomy. The presence or absence of an arterial pulse is not an accurate indicator of compartment pressures. Permanent damage may occur within 6 to 12 hr of onset.

chapter 7

EYE CARE

MYDRIATICS AND MIOTICS

Generic Name	Brand Name
Mydriatics Dilate pupils. Labels have *red* writing.	
Parasympathomimetics: Paralyze ciliary muscles as well as dilate	
Atropine sulfate	Isopto Atropine
Cyclopentolate	Cyclogyl
Homatropine hydrobromide	Homatrocel
	Isopto Homatropine
Physostigmine salicylate	Eserine
Tropicamide	Mydriacyl
Sympathomimetics	
Epinephrine	Adrenaline
	Epinephrine Biturate
Phenylephrine	Neo-Synephrine HCl
Miotics Constrict pupils. Labels have *green* writing.	
Acetazolamide	Diamox
Carbachol	Carcholin
	Doryl
	Isopto Carbachol
	P.V. Carbachol
Echothiophate iodide	Phospholine Iodide
Isoflurophate	Floropryl
Pilocarpine	Isopto Carpine
	Pilocar
	P.V. Carpine Liquifilm

INTRAOCULAR PRESSURE

With a Schiøtz tonometer, the normal reading is 11 to 22 mm Hg. The tonometer measures how much it indents the eyeball. The higher the pressure in the eyeball, the lower the reading on the tonometer. High intraocular pressure would give a reading of less than 11 mm Hg.

chapter 8

TOXIC INGESTIONS

chapter 8: **TOXIC INGESTIONS** 91

TOXIC DOSAGES

Acetaminophen: More than 140 mg/kg
Aspirin: More than 150 mg/kg
Iron: More than 20 mg/kg

TOXIC SERUM DRUG LEVELS[a,b]

Drug	Toxic Levels	Time Interval
Acetaminophen	>150 µg/ml	4 hr
Alcohol	>0.1 g/dl (legally intoxicated in most states)	—
Carbon monoxide	>10% of total hemoglobin	—
Digitoxin	>25 µg/ml	—
Digoxin	>2.5 µg/ml	—
Phenytoin	>20 µg/ml	—
Dyphylline	>20 µg/ml	—
Ibuprofen	>150 µg/ml	4 hr
Iron	>135 µg/ml	—
Iron binding capacity, total	<280 µg/ml	—
Lidocaine	>5 µg/ml	—
Lithium	>2.0 mEq/liter	—
Methanol	>50 µg/ml	—
Methemoglobin	>1.5% of total hemoglobin	—
Phenobarbital	>40 µg/ml	—
Procainamide	>12 µg/ml	—
Quinidine	>6 µg/ml	—
Salicylate	>250 µg/ml	6 hr
Theophylline	>20 µg/ml	—
Valproic acid	>200 µg/ml	—

[a] Courtesy of J. C. Calvanese, M.D., F.A.C.E.P., A.B.M.T.
[b] Some values may vary in different institutions.

TOXICITY NOMOGRAMS

Acetaminophen. From Rumack BH, Matthew H. Acetaminophen poisoning and toxicity. *Pediatrics* 1975; 55: 873.

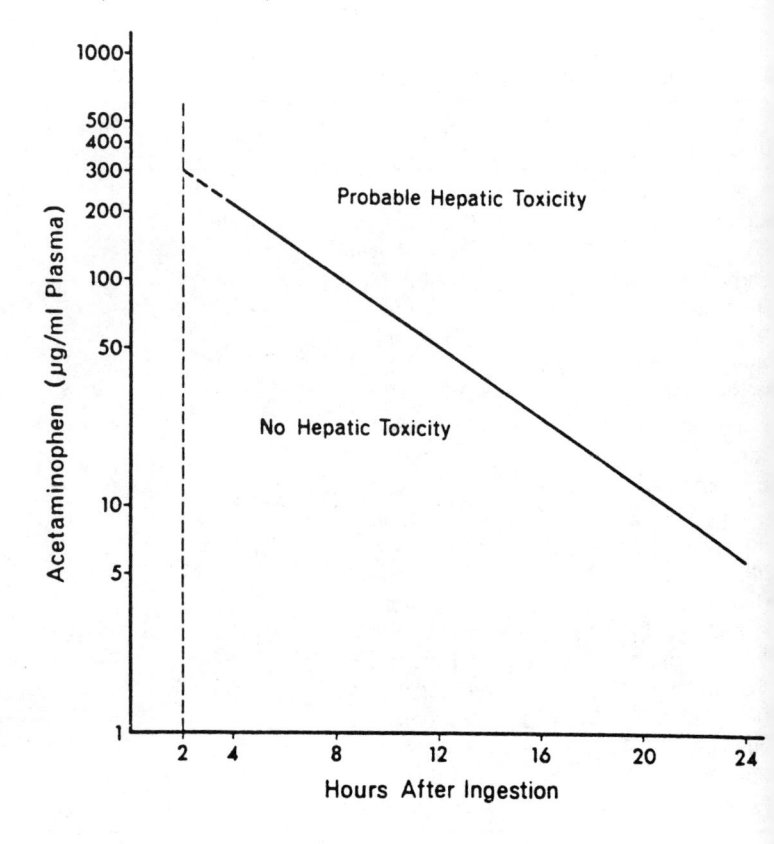

chapter **8: TOXIC INGESTIONS** 93

Ibuprofen. From Hall AH, Smolinske SC, Conrad FL, Wruk KM. et al. Ibuprofen overdose: 126 cases. Ann Emerg Med 1986; 15: 1309.

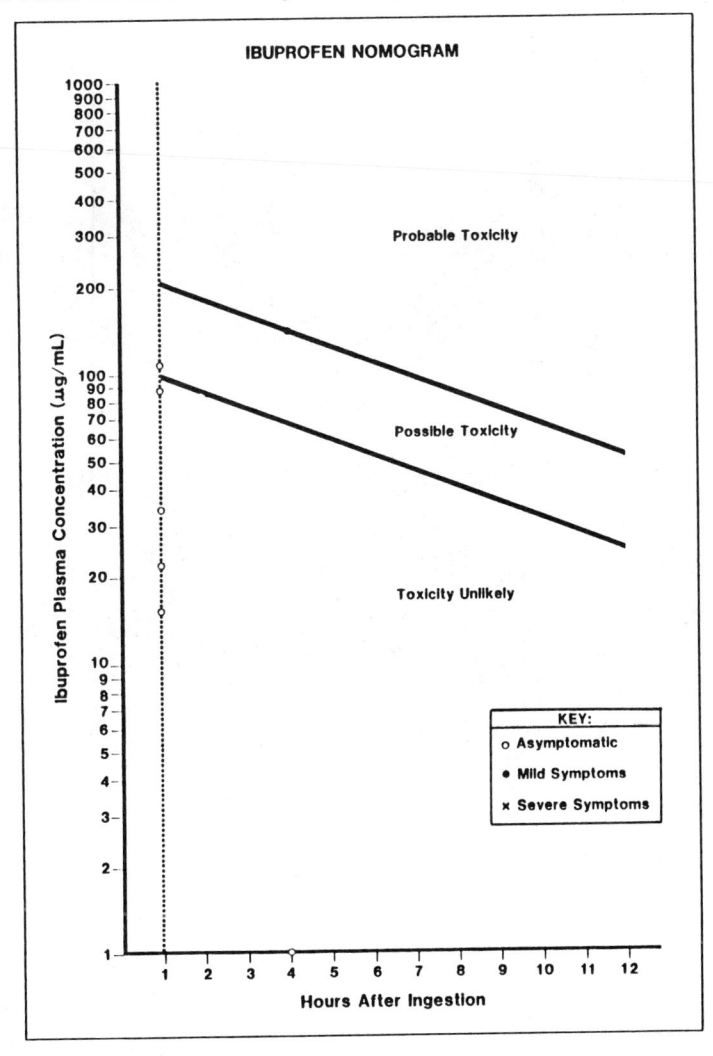

IBUPROFEN NOMOGRAM

Probable Toxicity

Possible Toxicity

Toxicity Unlikely

Ibuprofen Plasma Concentration (μg/mL)

Hours After Ingestion

KEY:
- ○ Asymptomatic
- ● Mild Symptoms
- × Severe Symptoms

Salicylate. Done AK. Salicylate intoxication: Significance of measurement of salicylate in blood in cases of acute ingestion. *Pediatrics* 1960; 26: 800.

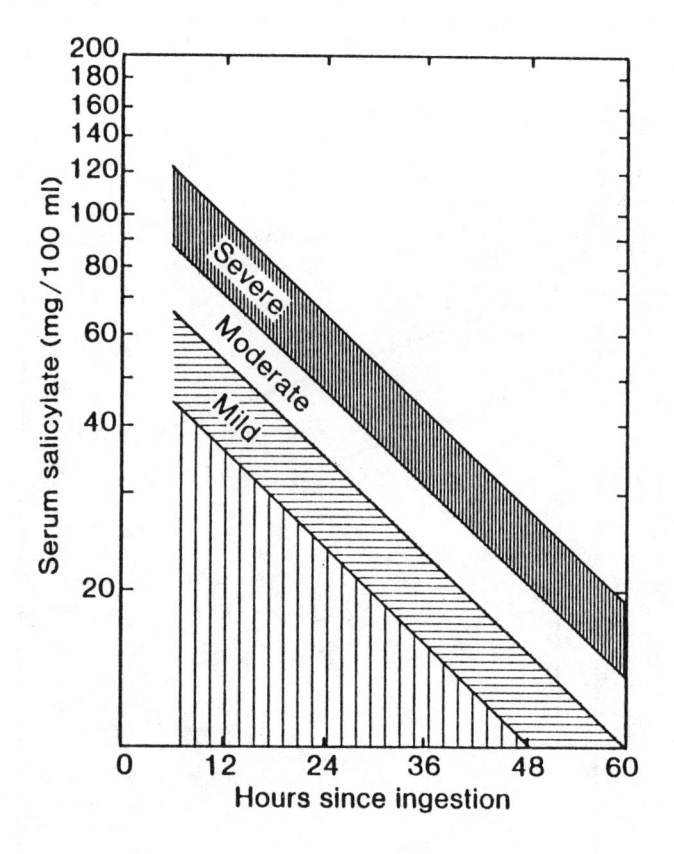

COMMON ANTIDOTES[a]

Poison	Local Antidote	Systemic Antidote
Acetaminophen	Activated charcoal (not to be used if acetylcysteine is to be given)	Acetylcysteine (Mucomyst)
Acids, corrosive	Dilute with water or milk	
Alkali, caustic	Dilute with water or milk, then give demulcent	
Alkaloids (coniine, quinine, strychnine, etc.)	Activated charcoal	
Amphetamines	Activated charcoal	
Anticholinergics	Activated charcoal	Physostigmine (controversial)
Anticholinesterases (organophosphates, neostigmine, physostigmine, pyridostigmine)	Activated charcoal	Atropine
Carbamates		Atropine
Antihistamines (see Anticholinergics)		
Arsenic (see Heavy Metal Chelation, this chapter)		
Atropine (see Anticholinergics)		
Belladonna alkaloids (see Anticholinergics)		
Bromides		Sodium or ammonium chloride

COMMON ANTIDOTES[a] *(cont.)*

Poison	Local Antidote	Systemic Antidote
Cadmium (see Heavy Metal Chelation, this chapter)		
Carbon monoxide		100% oxygen inhalation, preferably hyperbaric
Cholinergic compounds (see Anticholinesterases)		
Copper (see Heavy Metal Chelation, this chapter)		
Detergents, cationic	Ordinary soap solution	
Digoxin or digitoxin (see Digibind Dosages, this chapter)		
Ethylene glycol (see Methanol)		
Fluoride	Calcium gluconate or lactate	Calcium gluconate
Gold (see Heavy Metal Chelation, this chapter)		
Heparin sodium		Protamine sulfate 1% solution
Hypochlorites (see Alkali, caustic)		
Iodine	Starch solution, 3–10%	
Iron	Sodium bicarbonate, 1–5% solution, preferably by lavage	Deferoxamine

COMMON ANTIDOTES[a] *(cont.)*

Poison	Local Antidote	Systemic Antidote
Isoniazid (INH)	Activated charcoal	Pyridoxine (vitamin B_6)
Lead (see Heavy Metal Chelation, this chapter)		
Mercury (see Heavy Metal Chelation, this chapter)		
Methanol		Ethanol
Methemoglobinemic agents (nitrites, chlorates, nitrobenzene)		Methylene blue
Narcotics	Activated charcoal	Naloxone
Nitrites (see Methemoglobinemic agents)		
Oxalate	Dilute with water or milk, then give calcium gluconate or lactate	Calcium gluconate
Phenol	Dilute with water or milk, then give activated charcoal, castor oil, or vegetable oil	
Phenothiazines (neuromuscular reactions only)		Diphenhydramine
Phosgene		Methenamine
Quaternary ammonium compounds (see Detergents, cationic)		

COMMON ANTIDOTES[a] (cont.)

Poison	Local Antidote	Systemic Antidote
Silver (see Heavy Metal Chelation, this chapter)	Normal saline lavage	
Thallium (see Heavy Metal Chelation, this chapter)	Activated charcoal may be given continuously to remove metal excreted via enterohepatic circulation	
Warfarin (Coumadin)		Vitamin K_1

DIGIBIND DOSAGES

40 mg (1 vial) of Digibind binds about 0.6 mg of digoxin or digitoxin. Recommended dose of Digibind is 800 mg (20 vials) if the quantity ingested is unknown or digoxin levels cannot be obtained.

Step 1: Calculate total body load (TBL).

If amount ingested is known:

For digoxin tablets or elixir, TBL = dose ingested × 0.80
For digitoxin or Lanoxicaps, TBL = dose ingested

If serum digoxin concentration (SDC) is known:
Digoxin:

$$TBL = \frac{(SDC)(5.6)(wt\ in\ kg)}{1000}$$

Digitoxin:

$$TBL = \frac{(SDC)(0.56)(wt\ in\ kg)}{1000}$$

Step 2: Calculate the number of vials needed.

$$\text{Digibind dose in number of vials} = \frac{TBL}{0.6}$$

Digibind is usually given over 30 min unless cardiac arrest is imminent.

CYANIDE POISONING[a]

Adult: Amyl nitrite inhalation (inhale for 15–30 sec every 60 sec) pending administration of 300 mg sodium nitrite (10 ml of a 3% solution) i.v. slowly (over 2–4 min); follow immediately with 12.5 g sodium thiosulfate (2.5–5 ml/min of 25% solution) i.v. slowly (over 10 min).

Children: As for adult, but sodium nitrite should not exceed recommended dose, because fatal methemoglobinemia may result.

CYANIDE POISONING (cont.)

Child's Hemoglobin, g	Initial Dose 3% Sodium Nitrite i.v., ml/kg (mg/kg)		Initial Dose 25% Sodium Thiosulfate i.v., m/kg
8	0.22	(6.6)	1.10
10	0.27	(8.7)	1.35
12	0.33	(10)	1.65
14	0.39	(11.6)	1.95

[a]Adapted From Fleisher G, Ludwig S. Textbook of pediatric emergency medicine. 2nd ed. Baltimore: Williams & Wilkins, 1988.

HEAVY METAL CHELATION[a]

Heavy Metal	Usual Chelator
Arsenic	BAL[b]
Cadmium	Satisfactory use not demonstrated
Copper	BAL, penicillamine
Gold	BAL
Lead	BAL, CaEDTA,[c] penicillamine
Mercury	BAL, penicillamine[d]
Silver	Satisfactory use not demonstrated
Thallium	Satisfactory use not demonstrated

[a]Adapted From Fleisher G, Ludwig S. Textbook of pediatric emergency medicine. 2nd ed. Baltimore: Williams & Wilkins, 1988:

[b]BAL (dimercaprol): 3–5 mg/kg deep i.m. every 4 hr for 2 days, every 4–6 hr for additional 2 days, then every 4–12 hr for up to 7 additional days.

[c]EDTA: 75 mg/kg every 24 hr deep i.m. or slow i.v. infusion given in 3–6 divided doses for up to 5 days; may be repeated for a second course after a minimum of 2 days; each course should not exceed a total of 500 mg/kg body weight.

[d]Penicillamine: 100 mg/kg/day (maximum, 1 g) p.o. in divided doses for up to 5 days; for long-term therapy, do not exceed 40 mg/kg/day.

chapter 9

BURN CARE

chapter **9: BURN CARE** 103

Rule of Nines.

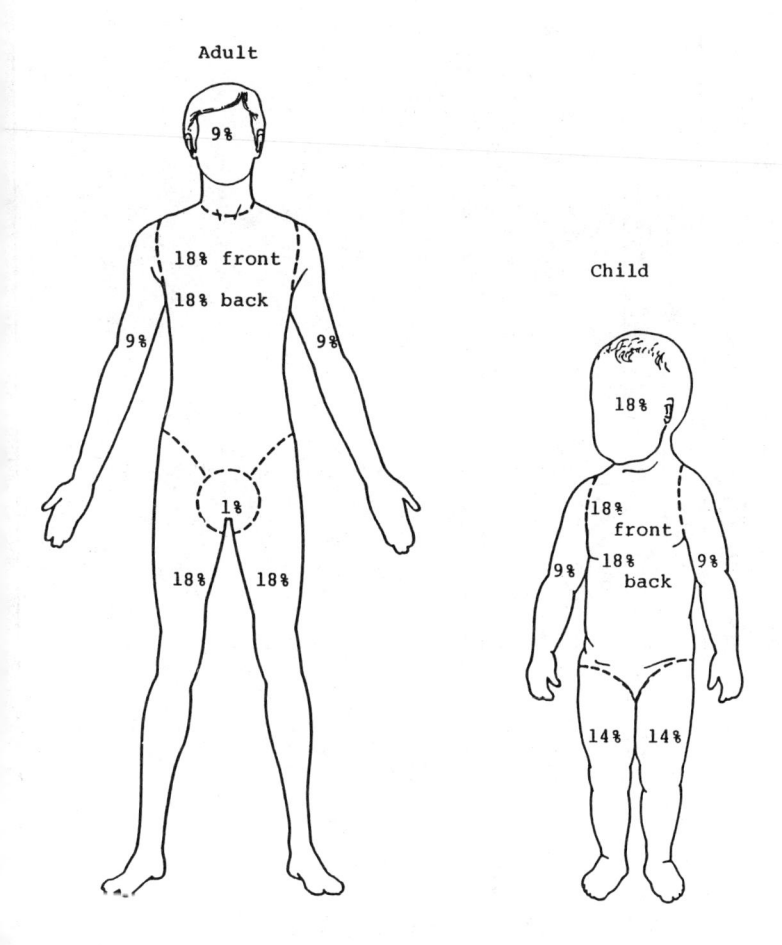

Adult

- 9% (head)
- 18% front
- 18% back
- 9% (each arm)
- 1% (perineum)
- 18% (each leg)

Child

- 18% (head)
- 18% front
- 18% back
- 9% (each arm)
- 14% (each leg)

LUND AND BROWDER BURN SURFACE CALCULATION

Burned Area	Age, yr 0–1	2–4	5–9	10–15	15+	% Second Degree	% Third Degree	% Total
Head	19	17	13	10	7			
Neck	2	2	2	2	2			
Anterior trunk	13	13	13	13	13			
Posterior trunk	13	13	13	13	13			
R buttock	2.5	2.5	2.5	2.5	2.5			
L buttock	2.5	2.5	2.5	2.5	2.5			
Genitalia	1	1	1	1	1			
R upper arm	4	4	4	4	4			
L upper arm	4	4	4	4	4			
R lower arm	3	3	3	3	3			
L lower arm	3	3	3	3	3			
R hand	2.5	2.5	2.5	2.5	2.5			
L hand	2.5	2.5	2.5	2.5	2.5			
R thigh	5.5	6.5	8.5	8.5	9.5			
L thigh	5.5	6.5	8.5	8.5	9.5			
R lower leg	5	5	5.5	6	7			
L lower leg	5	5	5.5	6	7			
R foot	3.5	3.5	3.5	3.5	3.5			
L foot	3.5	3.5	3.5	3.5	3.5			
					Totals			_____

FLUID REPLACEMENT FORMULAS

Formula	Day 1		Day 2	
	Crystalloid	Colloid	Crystalloid	Colloid
Parkland (Baxter)	Lactated Ringer's injection, 4 ml/kg per % body surface area burned	None	D5W, 2 liters/24 hr	40–60% of circulating volume
Modified Brooks	Lactated Ringer's injection, 2 ml/kg per % body surface area burned	None	Dextrose in saline, or normal saline to maintain adequate urine output	0.3 ml/kg per % body surface area burned
Evans	Normal saline, 1 ml/kg per % body surface area burned *plus* D5W, 2 liters/24 hr	1 ml/kg per % body surface area burned	One-half of first 24-hr requirement *plus* D5W, 2 liters/24 hr	One-half of first 24-hr requirement

chapter 10

PEDIATRICS

NORMAL VITAL SIGNS FOR INFANTS AND CHILDREN

Age	Pulse Range, per min[a]	Respiratory Range, per min[a]
Newborn	85–200	30–40
1 week–3 mo	85–160	30–40
3 mo–2 yr	100–190	28–34
4 yr	90–100	24–30
6 yr	80–90	22–28
8 yr	80–86	20–26
10 yr	76–84	20–24
12 yr	74–80	18–24

[a]These ranges are very rough estimates and should not be taken as absolute.

AVERAGE WEIGHT AND HEIGHT FOR INFANTS AND CHILDREN

Inches	cm	Weight, kg
18.0 – 20.5	46.0 – 52.0	3
20.5 – 22.25	52.0 – 56.5	4
22.25 – 23.75	56.5 – 60.5	5
23.75 – 25.25	60.5 – 64.0	6
25.25 – 26.5	64.0 – 67.5	7
26.5 – 28.25	67.5 – 71.5	8
28.25 – 29.75	71.5 – 75.5	9
29.75 – 31.5	75.5 – 80.0	10
31.5 – 33.5	80.0 – 85.0	11
33.5 – 35.5	85.0 – 90.0	12
35.5 – 37.0	90.0 – 94.0	13
37.0 – 38.5	94.0 – 98.0	14
38.5 – 40.0	98.0 – 101.5	15
40.0 – 41.25	101.5 – 104.5	16
41.25 – 42.5	104.5 – 107.5	17
42.5 – 43.5	107.5 – 110.5	18

AVERAGE WEIGHT AND HEIGHT FOR INFANTS AND CHILDREN *(cont.)*

Inches	cm	Weight, kg
43.5 – 44.75	110.5 – 113.5	19
44.75 – 46.0	113.5 – 117.0	20
46.0 – 48.0	117.0 – 122.0	22
48.0 – 49.75	122.0 – 126.0	24
49.75 – 51.25	126.0 – 130.0	26
51.25 – 52.75	130.0 – 134.0	28
52.75 – 53.75	134.0 – 136.5	30
53.75 – 55.0	136.5 – 140.0	32

EQUIPMENT GUIDELINES ACCORDING TO AGE AND WEIGHT[a,b]

Equipment	Premie (1–2.5 kg)	Neonate (2.5–4.0 kg)	6 mo (7.0 kg)	1–2 yr (10–12 kg)	5 yr (16–18 kg)	8–10 yr (24–30 kg)
Airway—oral	Infant (00)	Infant/small (0)	Small (1)	Small (2)	Medium (3)	Medium/large (4/5)
Breathing						
Self-inflating bag	Infant	Infant	Child	Child	Child	Child/adult
O_2 ventilation mask	Premature	Newborn	Infant/child	Child	Child	Small adult
Endotracheal tube	2.5–3.0 (uncuffed)	3.0–3.5 (uncuffed)	3.5–4.0 (uncuffed)	4.0–4.5 (uncuffed)	5.0–5.5 (uncuffed)	5.5–6.5 (cuffed)
Laryngoscope blade	0 (straight)	1 (straight)	1 (straight)	1–2 (straight)	2 (straight or curved)	2–3
Suction/stylet	6–8/6	8/6	8–10/6	10/6	14/14	14/14
Circulation						
BP cuff	Newborn	Newborn	Infant	Child	Child	Child/adult
Venous access						
Angiocath	22–24	22–24	22–24	20–22	18–20	16–20
Butterfly needle	25	23–25	23–25	23	20–23	18–21
Intracath	—	—	19	19	16	14
Arm board	6 in	6 in	6–8 in	8 in	8–15 in	15 in

EQUIPMENT GUIDELINES ACCORDING TO AGE AND WEIGHT[a,b] (cont.)

			Age (50th percentile weight)			
Equipment	Premie (1–2.5 kg)	Neonate (2.5–4.0 kg)	6 mo (7.0 kg)	1–2 yr (10–12 kg)	5 yr (16–18 kg)	8–10 yr (24–30 kg)
Orogastric tube	5	5–8	8	10	10–12	14–18
Chest tube	10–14	12–18	14–20	14–24	20–32	28–38

[a]From *Textbook of Pediatric Advanced Life Support*. American Heart Association

[b]**Foley catheter sizes:**
3–7 kg—5–8 Fr
8–11 kg—10 Fr
12–14 kg—10 Fr
15–24 kg—10–12 Fr
25–40 kg—12 Fr

PEDIATRIC CRASH DRUG AND DEFIBRILLATION DOSAGES

Defibrillation: 2 J/kg

Drug	How Supplied	Dosage
Epinephrine hydrochloride	1:10,000 (0.1 mg/ml)	0.01 mg/kg (0.1 ml/kg)
Sodium bicarbonate	1 mEq/ml (8.4% solution)	1 mEq/kg (1 ml/kg)
Atropine sulfate	0.1 mg/ml	0.02 mg/kg (0.2 ml/kg)
Calcium chloride	100 mg/ml (10% solution)	20 mg/kg (0.2 ml/kg)
Glucose	0.5 g/ml D50W	0.5–1 g/kg (Dilute 1:1 with water: 2–4 ml/kg)
Lidocaine hydrochloride	10 mg/ml (1%) or 20 mg/ml (2%)	1 mg/kg
Bretylium tosylate	50 mg/ml	5 mg/kg (0.1 ml/kg)

PEDIATRIC INTRAVENOUS DRUG CONCENTRATIONS

Drug	Mixture	Concentration	Suggested Starting Dose
Dopamine (40 mg/ml)	60 mg (1.5 ml)/100 ml D5W	600 µg/ml	0.5–1.0 ml/kg/hr = 5–10 µg/kg/min
Epinephrine (1:10,000)	0.6 mg (3 ml)/100 ml D5W	6 µg/ml	1 ml/kg/hr = 0.1 µg/kg/min
Isoproterenol (1:5,000)	0.6 mg (0.6 ml)/100 ml D5W	6 µg/ml	1 ml/kg/hr = 0.1 µg/kg/min
Lidocaine (4%)	120 mg (3 ml)/100 ml D5W	1200 µg/ml	1 ml/kg/hr = 20 µg/kg/min

(*cont. on page 114*)

PEDIATRIC INTRAVENOUS DRUG CONCENTRATIONS (cont.)

Drug	Mixture	Concentration	Suggested Starting Dose
Nitroprusside	6 mg/100 ml D5W	60 µg/ml	1 ml/kg/hr = 1 µg/kg/min

FORMULA FOR INTRAVENOUS VOLUME REPLACEMENT

Assess for signs of hypovolemic shock
(Tachycardia, pallor, decreased level of consciousness, delayed capillary refill, low blood pressure)

↓

20 ml/kg Ringer's lactate solution
given rapidly (less than 20 min)

↓

Reassess

↓

If signs of hypovolemic shock remain,
Additional 20 ml/kg crystalloid or colloid

↓

Children often require 40–60 ml/kg

MODIFIED INFANT COMA SCORE[a]

Activity	Best Response	Score
Eye opening	Spontaneous	4
	To speech	3
	To pain	2
	None	1
Verbal	Coos, babbles	5
	Irritable cries	4
	Cries to pain	3
	Moans to pain	2
	None	1
Motor	Normal spontaneous movements	6
	Withdraws from touch	5
	Withdraws from pain	4
	Abnormal flexion	3
	Abnormal extension	2
	None	1
	Total	____

[a]From Selbst SM, Torrey SB: Pediatric emergency medicine for the house officer. Baltimore: Williams & Wilkins, 1988: 67.

COMMON PEDIATRIC LABORATORY VALUES

Laboratory values vary in different hospitals. Check the normal value given for adults to see that it coincides with that used at your hospital.

Acid phosphatase	
Newborns	7.4–19.4 IU/ml
2–13 yr	6.4–15.2 IU/ml
Adults	0.2–11 IU/ml
Alkaline phosphatase	
Newborns	20–266 IU/liter
1 mo–1yr	50–260 IU/liter
1–2 yr	146–477 IU/liter
2–6 yr	70–160 IU/liter
6–10 yr	45–273 IU/liter
Adolescents	56–253 IU/liter
Adults	13–40 IU/liter
Calcium	
Newborns	7.0–12.0 mg/dl
Children	8–11.0 mg/dl
Adults	8.5–11 mg/dl
Copper	
0–6 mo	70 µg/dl
6 mo–5 yr	27–153 µg/dl
5–17 yr	94–234 µg/dl
Adults	70–155 µg/dl
Creatine phosphokinase	
Newborns	30–100 U/liter
Children	15–50 U/liter
Adults	5–10 U/liter

(*cont. on page 117*)

COMMON PEDIATRIC LABORATORY VALUES *(cont.)*

Creatinine (serum)
    1–18 mo   0.2–0.5 mg/dl
    2–12 yr   0.3–0.8 mg/dl
    13–20 yr   0.5–1.2 mg/dl
    Adults   0.8–1.5 mg/dl
Iron Binding Capacity
    Newborn   59–175 μg/dl
    1 mo to adult   250–400 μg/dl
Magnesium
    Newborns   1.52–2.33 mEq/liter
    Children   1.4–1.9 mEq/liter
    Adults   1.3–2.5 mEq/liter
Phosphorus
    Newborn   4.0–10.5 mg/dl
    1 yr   4.0–6.8 mg/dl
    5 yr   3.6–6.5 mg/dl
    Adult   3–4.5 mg/dl
Proteins (total)
    Newborns   5–7.1 g/dl
    1–3 mo   4.7–7.4 g/dl
    3–12 mo   5–7.5 g/dl
    1–15 yr   6.5–8.6 g/dl
    Adults   6–8.4 g/dl
Transaminase (SGOT)
    1–3 days   16–74 U/liter
    3 days–6 mo   20–43 U/liter
    6 mo–1 yr   16–35 U/liter
    1 yr–5 yr   6–30 U/liter
    5 yr–adults   19–28 U/liter
    Adults   Female: 7–34 U/liter
                                         Male: 8–16 U/liter

HEMATOLOGY

Age	Hgb, g/100 ml	HCT, %	MCV, fl	MCHC, gm/dl RBC	Reticulocyte, %	WBC per ml × 100 range (avg)	% Neutrophils
Newborns	16.8–21.2	57–68	110–128	29.7–33.5	1.8–4.6	7–35 (18)	45–85
3–5 mo	10.4–12.2	33	80–96	31.8–36.2	0.4–1	6–17 (10)	30–50
6–11 mo	11.8	35	77	33	0.7–2.3	6–16 (10)	30–50
1 yr	11.2	35	78	32	0.6–1.7	6–15 (10)	30–50
2–10 yr	12.8	37	80	34	0.5–1	7–13 (9)	35–60
11–15 yr	13.4	39	82	34	0.5–1	5–12 (8.5)	40–60
Adults							
Males	16 ± 2	47 ± 7			0.8–2.5		
			82–101	31.5–36		4.3–10 (7)	25–62
Females	14 ± 2	42 ± 5			0.3–4.1		

APGAR SCORING

Score each category, then total those numbers. Scoring is done at 1 min and at 5 min after birth.

Sign	Score 0	Score 1	Score 2
Heart rate	Absent	< 100/min	>100/min
Respirations	Absent	Slow, irregular	Good, crying
Muscle tone	Limp	Some flexion	Active motion
Reflex irritability (catheter in nares)	No response	Grimace	Cough or sneeze
Color	Blue or pale	Pink body with blue limbs	Completely pink

IMMUNIZATION SCHEDULE

Age	Immunizations	Comments
2 mo	DTP, OPV	Can be early as 2 wk if endemic
4 mo	DTP, OPV	2-mo interval desired for OPV to avoid interference with previous dose
6 mo	DTP, (OPV)	OPV is optional (may be given in areas with high risk)
15 mo	MMR	Tuberculin testing may be done
18 mo	DTP, OPV	DTP should be 6–12 mo after first dose. OPV may be given at same time as MMR

(*cont. on page 120*)

IMMUNIZATION SCHEDULE *(cont.)*

Age	Immunizations	Comments
24 mo	HBPV	
4–6 yr	DTP, OPV	At or before school entry, up to 7th birthday
14–16 yr	dT	Repeat every 10 yr through lifetime

DTP—Diptheria and tetanus toxoids with pertussis vaccine.
dT—Adult diphtheria toxoid (reduced dose) and tetanus toxoid (full dose).
HBPV—*Haemophilus influenzae* b polysaccharide vaccine.
MMR—Live measles, mumps, rubella viruses in a vaccine.
OPV—Oral poliovirus vaccine.

ACETAMINOPHEN DOSAGES[a]

15 mg/kg or 7 mg/lb
Every 4 to 6 hrs as needed
Do not give more than 5 doses a day

Weight, lb	Drops,[b] ml	Liquiprin Drops,[c] droppers	Elixir or Liquid,[d] tsp	Children's Tablets,[e] tablets	Junior Tablets,[f] tablets
6–11	0.4–0.8	½–1	¼–½		
12–17	0.8–1.2	1–1½	½–¾		
18–23	1.2–1.6	1½–2	¾–1	1½–2	
24–35	1.6–2.4	2–3	1–1½	2–3	1–1½
36–47	2.4–3.2	3–4	1½–2	3–4	1½–2
48–59	3.2–4	4–5	2–2½	4–5	2–2½
60–71	4.0–4.8	5–6	2½–3	5–6	2½–3
72–95	4.8–6.4	6–7	3–4	6–7	3–4

[a]Courtesy of Washoe Medical Center, Reno, Nevada.
[b]100 mg/ml.
[c]80 mg/dropper.
[d]80 mg/½ tsp (2.5 ml).
[e]80 mg/tablet.
[f]160 mg/tablet.

… # appendix A

ABBREVIATIONS

appendix A: ABBREVIATIONS

ACLS Advanced cardiac life support
Apr April
Aug August
C Centigrade
Dec December
D5W 5% dextrose in water
dl deciliter
F Fahrenheit
Feb February
Fr French
g gram
gr grain
gtt drops
HCT hematocrit
Hg mercury
Hgb hemoglobin
hr hour
i.m. intramuscular
i.v. intravenous
IU international unit
Jan January
Jul July
Jun June
kg kilogram
lb pound
µg microgram
µl microliter
Mar March
MCHC mean corpuscular hemoglobin concentration
MCL modified chest lead
MCV mean corpuscular volume
mEq milliequivalent
mg milligram
min minute
ml milliliter
mm millimeter
Nov November
Oct October
p.o. by mouth (per os)
prn as occasion arises (pro re nata)
pt patient
RBC red blood cell
s.c. subcutaneous
Sep September
sltn solution

tsp teaspoon

U unit

WBC white blood cell

wt weight

appendix B

HEALTH CARE–RELATED TELEPHONE NUMBERS

appendix B: HEALTH CARE—RELATED TELEPHONE NUMBERS

AIDS Information Line
(800) 342-AIDS
Centers for Disease Control
Atlanta, GA 30333

Al-Anon Family Group Headquarters
(800) 344-2666
1372 Broadway
New York, NY 10018-0862

Alzheimer's Disease and Related Disorders Association (ADRDA)
(800) 621-0379 (outside IL)
(800) 572-6037 (within IL)
70 E. Lake St. #600
Chicago, IL 60601

American Academy of Facial Plastic and Reconstructive Surgery
(800) 332-FACE (USA)
(800) 523-FACE (Canada)
1101 Vermont Ave., NW,
Suite 304
Washington, DC 20005

American Academy of Pediatrics (AAP)
(800) 421-0589 (within IL)
(800 433-9016 (outside IL)
141 NW Point Rd.
P.O. Box 927
Elk Grove, IL 60007

American Association of Critical Care Nurses (AACN)
(714) 644-9310
One Civic Plaza
Newport Beach, CA 92660

American Cleft Palate Educational Foundation
(800) 242-5338 (outside PA)
(800) 232-5338 (within PA)
1218 Grandview Ave.
Pittsburgh, PA 15211

American College of Emergency Physicians
(214) 550-0911
P.O. Box 619911
Dallas, TX 75261-9911

American Diabetes Association
(800) 232-3472
1660 Duke St.
Alexandria, VA 22314

American Foundation for the Blind
(800) 232-5463
15 W. 16th St.
New York, NY 10011

American Heart Association
(214) 748-7212
7320 Greenville Ave.
Dallas, TX 75231

American Kidney Fund
(800) 638-8299 (outside MD)
(800) 492-8361 (within MD)
6110 Executive Blvd.,
Suite 1010
Rockville, MD 20852

American Liver Foundation
(800) 223-0179
998 Pompton Ave.
Cedar Grove, NJ 07009

American Nurses Association
(816) 474-5720
2420 Pershing Rd.
Kansas City, MO 64108

American Trauma Society
(800) 556-7890 (outside MD)
P.O. Box 13526
Baltimore, MD 21203

Better Hearing Institute
(800) 424-8576
Box 1840
Washington, DC 20013

Bulimia Anorexia Self-Help (BASH)
(800) BASH-STL
6125 Clayton Ave., Suite 215
St. Louis, MO 63139-3295

Cancer Information Service
(800) 4-CANCER
(800) 524-1234 (within Hawaii)
(800) 638-6070 (within Alaska)
Office of Cancer
Communications, NCI, NIH
Bldg. 31, Rm. 10A24
9000 Rockville Pike
Bethesda, MD 20892

Consumer Product Safety Commission (CPSC)
(800) 638-2772 (Consumer Hotline)
Washington, DC 20207

Cystic Fibrosis Foundation
(800) 344-4823
6931 Arlington Rd.
Bethesda, MD 20814

Emergency Nurses Association
(312) 649-0297
230 East Ohio, Suite 600
Chicago, IL 60611

Endometriosis Association
(800) 992-ENDO
P.O. Box 92187
Milwaukee, WI 53202

Epilepsy Foundation of America
(800) EFA-1000 (outside MD)
(301) 459-3700 (within MD)
4351 Garden City Dr., Suite 406
Landover, MD 20785

Family Survival Project for Brain-Damaged Adults
(800) 445-8106
44 Page St., Suite 600
San Francisco, CA 94102

Guide Dog Foundation for the Blind
(800) 548-4337
371 E. Jericho Turnpike
Smithtown, NY 11787

Health Resources and Services Administration
Bureau of Health Maintenance Organizations and Resources
Office of Health Facilities
(800) 492-0359
5600 Fishers Lane
Rockville, MD 20857

Juvenile Diabetes Foundation
(800) 223-1138
432 Park Ave., S., 16th Floor
New York, NY 10016

appendix B: HEALTH CARE—RELATED TELEPHONE NUMBERS

Lupus Foundation of America
(800) 558-0121
1717 Massachusetts Ave., NW,
Suite 203
Washington, DC 20036

Medic Alert Foundation International
(800) 344-3226 (outside CA)
(209) 668-3333 (within CA)
2323 Colorado
Turlock, CA 95381-1009

Missing Children Help Center
(800) USA-KIDS (outside FL)
(813) 623-5437 (within FL)
410 Ware Blvd., #400
Tampa, FL 33619

National Abortion Federation
(800) 772-9100
900 Pennsylvania Ave., SE
Washington, DC 20003

National Association for Hearing and Speech Action
(800) 638-8453
10801 Rockville Pike
Rockville, MD 20852

National Association for Sickle Cell Disease
(800) 421-8453
4221 Wilshire Blvd., Suite 360
Los Angeles, CA 90010-3505

National Asthma Center
(800) 222-5864
3800 E. Colfax Ave.
Denver, CO 80206

National Center for Missing and Exploited Children
(800) 843-5678
1835 K Street NW, Suite 700
Washington, DC 20006

National Child Safety Council
(800) 222-1464
P.O. Box 1368
Jackson, MI 49204

National Cocaine Hotline
(800) 262-2463
Fair Oaks Hospital
19 Prospect St.
Summit, NJ 07901

National Council on Alcoholism
(800) NCA-CALL
12 West 21st St., Suite 700
New York, NY 10010

National Gay Task Force
(800) 221-7044 (Information on AIDS)
80 5th Ave., Suite 1601
New York, NY 10011

National Head Injury Foundation
(800) 444-6443
333 Turnpike Rd.
Southboro, MA 01772

National Headache Foundation
(800) 843-2256 (outside IL)
(800) 523-8858 (within IL)
5252 North Western Ave.
Chicago, IL 60625

National Health Information Center
(800) 336-4797 (outside MD)
P.O. Box 1133
Washington, DC 20013-1133

National Multiple Sclerosis Society
(800) 624-8236
205 E. 42nd St.
New York, NY 10017

National Pesticide Telecommunications Network
(800) 858-7378
3601 4th St.
Lubbock, TX 79430

National Reye's Syndrome Foundation, Inc.
(800) 233-7393 (outside OH)
(800) 231-7393 (within OH)
P.O. Box 829
Bryan, OH 43506

National Runaway Switchboard
(800) 231-6946 (outside TX)
(800) 392-3552 (within TX)
P.O. Box 12428
Austin, TX 78711

National Spinal Cord Injury Association
(800) 962-9629
149 California St.
Newton, MA 02158

National Sudden Death Syndrome Foundation
(800) 221-SIDS (outside MD)
(301) 459-3388 (within MD)
8200 Professional Pl., Suite 104
Landover, MD 20785

North American Nursing Diagnosis Association
(314) 577-8954
3525 Caroline St.
St. Louis, MO 63104

PMS Access
(Information on premenstrual syndrome)
(800) 237-4666
P.O. Box 9326
Madison, WI 53715

Parents Anonymous
(800) 421-0353 (outside CA)
(800) 352-0386 (within CA)
7120 Franklin Ave.
Los Angeles, Ca 90046

Y-Me Breast Cancer Support Program
(800) 221-2141
1757 Ridge Rd.
Homewood, IL 60430